VIRUSES
AND THEIR METHODS OF
IDENTIFICATION

F ESTUS   D. A DU

Order this book online at www.trafford.com
or email orders@trafford.com

Most Trafford titles are also available at major online book retailers.

Printed in the United States of America.

ISBN: 978-1-4269-5667-6 (sc)
ISBN: 978-1-4269-5668-3 (e)

Trafford rev. 03/01/2011

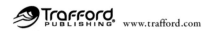

www.trafford.com

North America & international
toll-free: 1 888 232 4444 (USA & Canada)
phone: 250 383 6864 • fax: 812 355 4082

DEDICATION

This book is dedicated to all my students, most of whom are also making their impact felt and contributing to the knowledge of virology in different parts of the world and to the memory of those Nigerian children who have lost their cherished lives to the cold hands of death, as a result of virus infection.

ACKNOWLEDGEMENT

I thank the Almighty God, the author of all knowledge and wisdom, for giving me the inspiration and strength to write this book. I thank my collaborators, Olen Kew, Mark Pallansch and Paul Rota of Centres for Disease Control and Prevention(CDC), Atlanta Georgia, USA where I learned most of the molecular techniques presented in the book. They provided me a comfortable working space for writing during my annual visits to CDC as a visiting researcher. I remember vividly that it was at my sitting desk at the CDC that I got the inspiration to start putting this book together. I thank the WHO for the permission to use some of the figures and sections of the WHO Polio Manual. I also thank the Yale University Press for permission to reproduce some pictures from Hsiungs Diagnostic Virology. I thank my family for their encouragement and belief in Daddy's effort to achieve. I thank Dr. Waidi Folorunso, who took the pains to read through the initial script and Professor Lekan Oyejide, for the final editing. Finally I thank both Mrs Adeagbo and Mrs Olanubi, for the typing and secretarial jobs on the book.

Contents

PART I
GENERAL PROPERTIES OF VIRUSES

PART II
DIAGNOSTIC METHODS FOR ISOLATING
AND IDENTIFYING VIRUSES

PART III
SPECIFIC VIRUS FAMILIES: CHARACTERISTICS, IDENTIICATION AND LABORATORY DIAGNOSIS

RNA VIRUSES

DNA VIRUSES

Figures

TABLE

FOREWORD

Professor Festus Adu has written an eminently readable book that presents in adequate detail, the basic principles of tropical virology and describes simple, optimised techniques for efficient diagnostic virology laboratory practice. Adu's considerable enthusiasm and passion for virology manifest clearly in the flowing pages of this well written tome. Given the paucity of locally written books on this and other specialty biomedical subjects, this volume is a significant and welcome contribution to the list of publications in the discipline, coming as it does from the experiences and perspective of an expert based in the tropics. Professor Adu's book is unpretentious but authoritative, reflecting his more than three decade experience first as a government research virologist in Vom, and subsequently, as consultant clinical virologist at the University of Ibadan, Nigeria. Adu wrote this book during his tenure at the College of Medicine when he served as Professor and Head of the Department of Virology and as Director of the WHO National Polio Laboratory, Ibadan. Thus, a significant proportion of the book derives from his lecture notes to medical and postgraduate students at Ibadan and from his research laboratory notes at the Department of Virology. It is little wonder then that aspects of the book read like a practitioners' guide to diagnostic virology and of understanding of the general as well as basic principles of virology. This is quite apt, of course, since the book is targeted at medical, veterinary and allied health students who need to take assigned virology courses, including wet labs; and to technical and research staff who are tasked with processing clinical samples for the detection of virus infections. No matter the background of the reader, the clear and concise writing style will be enjoyed by all. Professor Adu introduces the reader to the discipline in a step-wise manner that is straightforward and easy to assimilate. The book deals at length with the various steps to optimise virus culture, isolation and identification, using routine and molecular techniques, the emphasis being on the important viruses of the tropics. Despite this simple approach, Adu has not skimped on explanations that help the student understand the more complex molecular basis of the pathogenesis of virus diseases and the role of molecular techniques in diagnostic virology. For those in need of even more detail, each chapter ends with suggested further readings selected from literature sources that can be accessed readily in many tropical country institutions as well as from popular internet web sites that allow free article downloads.

The first part of the book is devoted to general virology. Here, Professor Adu describes the properties and nature of viruses, with some well deserved emphasis on quality assurance and safety procedures in virology laboratories. This first section refocuses our attention on the growing impact of tropical virus infections including HIV, polio and reiterates the need for improved laboratory infrastructure to support disease surveillance in the affected countries. In making the case for surveillance as a worthwhile endeavour for the ultimate control of tropical virus infections, Adu's book succeeds remarkably in drawing the reader's attention to the enormous need for more diagnostic virology capabilities in those countries where these diseases are still major scourges of animal and human health.

In the second part of the book, Professor Adu describes various laboratory tests for the identification and diagnosis of viral diseases. This section deals at length with the various steps to optimise virus culture, isolation and identification, using routine and molecular techniques. Methods for the detection and identification of human and animal viruses presented include: protein based (ELISA and Western immunoblotting) and nucleic acid (PCR, RT-PCR, qPCR and dot-blot hybridization) techniques. The underlying principles of these techniques are simplified and presented in well-constructed outlines and "menus" that should help beginners and experienced technicians alike achieve optimal results. This section represents a major strength of the book, deriving as it does from the author's laboratory experiences at Ibadan and from his long term collaborative research activities at the Centers for Disease Control (CDC) in Atlanta, USA.

The third and final part of the book represents the standard didactic virology text section in that it deals with individual virus families. Individual properties and characteristics of the various viruses are described and type(s) of laboratory tests required for their recognition and diagnosis are presented. Although the section focuses on the major families of viruses, the emphasis again is on those of relative importance in the tropics.

In conclusion, Professor Adu has managed to provide in this volume, a comprehensive book of tropical medical virology that is both readable and affordable. In my opinion, this book has the potential to become a classic. I, therefore, warmly recommend it to all present and future students of virology, especially those with an interest in tropical diseases.

Adelekan Oyejide, DVM, PhD, Diplomate ACVP.
Principal Research Pathologist, Merck Inc., Summit, NJ, USA
Formerly, Scientific Director, Pathology, Allergan Inc, Irvine CA, USA.
Formerly, Professor/Head, Dept of Veterinary Pathology, University of Ibadan, Nigeria.

PREFACE

The discipline of virology started as a branch of pathology which is the study of diseases. Unfortunately the burden of diseases caused by viruses is enormous in the African continent. I would remember in 1999 during my attendance at an international conference on epidemiology in the US, nearly all those who spoke would point to one or two countries in Africa as the source of one virus or the other. I could not but ask why Mother Nature decided to bury so many of the viruses under the soil of Africa.

Viruses are of so much ecological, health and evolutionary importance. They have caused more death than all the world wars combined. The appearance of any novel virus, especially the fast spreading types, will almost surely cause a global stampede among the world communities. It is therefore pertinent that for effective diagnosis, control, prevention and rapid response to outbreaks, the study of virology should be paramount in our educational institutions-intermediate, undergraduate and postgraduate levels. Although many excellent books have been written on virology, very few have been written by Nigerian authors. This was the driving motivation for me to write this book as part of my experience of 37 years as a research-, teaching- and laboratory-virologist both at the National Veterinary Research Institute Vom, Plateau State and at the College of Medicine, University of Ibadan, Ibadan Nigeria.

The book is divided into three parts. The first part is a general aspect that describes the nature of viruses, bio-safety, specimen collection and processing and quality assurance. The second part describes the diagnostic methods for isolating and identifying viruses. The various laboratory tests used for identification and final diagnosis of these viruses are described in details and in practical terms. In this part also, I have devoted a chapter to the technology of monoclonal antibody production because of the important role they play in those specific tests needed for the identification, typing and diagnosis of viruses. The third part describes the specific virus families, their characteristics, identification and laboratory diagnosis starting with the RNA viruses.

The Global Polio Laboratory Network has developed a large technical expertise and infrastructure, the lesson and experience of which can be easily applied to the diagnosis and surveillance of other important viral diseases. With my experience as the Director of the Ibadan National Polio Laboratory for fifteen years, I have therefore taken some time to describe the structure of the Global Poliovirus Laboratory Network and some of the tests used for polio and enterovirus diagnosis.

The book is both theoretical and practical, meant both for those in lecture halls and those on the bench. It is my hope that the book will be attractive to medical students, veterinary students, undergraduate and postgraduate students of virology and microbiology, practising physicians, laboratory technologists and nurses as well as the "bankers" who were asking me "What is Virology?" when in 1996 I went cap-in- hand sourcing for fund to run our Department of Virology when I assumed the headship of the Department in 1996.

I have cited some important references in the book for further reading by the reader who may want more information on a specific topic.

F.D. Adu

PART I

GENERAL PROPERTIES OF VIRUSES

CHAPTER 1

Introduction

The discipline Virology began as a branch of pathology, the study of diseases. Long after the agents of some important diseases were recognised, it was quite clear to pathologists that there were other infectious diseases of man for which neither bacterium nor protozoa was incriminated. The discovery of the membrane filter, which had the ability of retaining the smallest bacteria or protozoa but will allow other infectious agents to pass through soon put this misunderstanding to rest. It was a German anatomist Jacob Henle who in 1840, first hypothesised the existence of infectious agents that was too small to be observed with the ordinary light microscope and were also capable of causing specific diseases. Although his hypothesis could not be accepted at that time, it took several other scientists – Pasteur, Koch, Lister Mayer, Ivanofski, Beijerinck, d'Herelle, Loeffler and Frosch from different countries, often working independent of each other for many years to come to a new concept of a filterable agent too small to be observed with the light microscope but able to cause disease by multiplying in living cells. It was then named *contagium vivum fluidum*. Loeffler and Frosch isolated the first filterable agent from an animal- the Foot and Mouth disease virus while Walter Reed (1901) recognised the first human filterable diseases causing agent – the Yellow Fever virus. Loeffler and Frosch in 1898 were able to transfer the Foot and Mouth disease of cattle from one animal to the other through a filtrate. Today, after many years of the study of the morphology and structure of these groups of infectious agents, viruses can be defined as microscopically minute, metabolically inert obligate intracellular infectious parasites which are unable to grow or reproduce outside host cells. The name virus (limy liquid or poison) became to be restricted to those agents that fulfilled the criteria of Mayers, Ivanosfki and Beijerinck. The viral particle usually refered to as a virion consists of a genetic material which can either be deoxyribonucleic acid (DNA) or ribonucleic acid (RNA) which are enclosed in a protective coat protein called capsid. Since their discovery, viruses have come to assume a very significant position in the pathology of many diseases of man and animals. They have even now been incriminated in such diseases that were once thought to be outside their influence where they may not be the direct cause but have been observed to aggravate or exacabate the disease conditions such as the role of some enteroviruses in development of heart disease and some respiratory viruses like influenza virus in the development and pathogenesis of asthma. Viruses have shaped the history and evolution of their hosts because of their parasitic nature. This group of microorganisms is of so much ecological, health and evolutionary importance because virtually all living organisms when studied carefully have been found to have one viral parasite. These very small microscopic organisms, regardless of their sizes exert significant forces on all forms of life, even including themselves. Viruses have caused more human death than all the world-wars combined. The medical consequences of human viral infections have altered the human history and have resulted in extraordinary efforts on the part of virologists to study, understand and eradicate these agents. With increase in technological know-how and availability of modern scientific equipments coupled with advent of new methodologies and the development of tissue culture, new viruses are discovered every year.

As important as viruses were to be recognised later as important causes of diseases, diagnostic virology was outside of the mainstream of clinical laboratory medicine. This was because virology laboratories depend on tissue culture and cell culture techniques, reagent were not always available and only very few viral infections could be treated. The tissue culture technique was unusually slow and expensive and so physicians were reluctant to rely in the procedures as a rapid means of instituting treatment or intervention.

Fortunately, all this has changed. Diagnostic virology is presently integrated into routine medical practice. The need for rapid intervention, that will lead to control and prevention as well as saving life have made this mandatory. Viral disease frontiers are expanding everyday as a result of a growing human population, increased travel between different parts of the world, and increased human entry into sylvan areas or possibly increased contact with wild animals harbouring viruses potentially capable of transmitting to humans (e.g., bush meat and HIV). This makes it possible for more people becoming infected by viral diseases. The advent of the human immunodeficiency virus (HIV) and acquired immunodeficiency syndrome (AIDS) pandemic have increased the pool of patients at the risk of serious opportunistic viral infections. The introduction of novel technologies like monoclonal antibodies, the polymerase chain reaction (PCR) and other nucleic acid amplification assays have greatly shortened the period of waiting for results of clinical samples. Better still is the recent discovery of the qualitative Real-Time polymerase chain reaction (qRT-PCR) methodology which makes PCR more practical and applicable for clinical laboratories. The number of antiviral drugs in the market today has increased tremendously. Laboratory-based diagnoses are needed to validate their activities.

All the above have facilitated the development of quantitative assays.

Today, multiple techniques are available for detecting viral infections. These include virus culture and detection of viral antigens, serology for detecting viral antibodies, methods for detecting nucleic acids and its components and methods for detection of viral infection in tissue. All these can be carried out in a number of clinical laboratories.

The various tests have become very important, especially in the treatment and management of immunocompromised patients,

patients with sexually transmitted diseases, acute respiratory diseases and gastrointestinal infections, hepatitis patients and a host of pediatric infections.

Laboratory tests are also very important tools for disease surveillance, especially in the recognition of potential new strains of viruses. Such tests are also very important in monitoring and directing immunisation programmes as well as in putting in place control programmes like the Global Polio Eradication Initiative (PEI) and mosquitoes or rodent control in arboviral infections.

Further Reading
1. d'Herelle F. *The bacteriophage and its behavior.* Baltimore Williams and Milkins 1926.

2. d'Herelle FH. *Sur un microbe invisible antagoniste.* Des bacilles dysenteriques C.R. Hebd séances Acad. Sci. Paris, 1921; 1: 72:99

3. Ivanofsky D. "Mosaic disease of the tobacco plant." *St Petersbourg Acad Imp Sci Bull. 1892: 35:67-70.*

4. Lwoff A. Siminovitch, L. Kjeldgaard N. "Induction de la lyse bacteriophagique de la totalite d'tune population microbionne lysogene." *C.R. Acad Sci Paris, 1950: 231: 190-191.*

5. Mayer A. "On the Mosaic disease of tobacco." Landum Versstnen 1886:32, 451-467

6. Pasteur L. "Methode pour prevenir l rage après morsure" *C.R. Acad Sci 1885: 101: 765-772.*

CHAPTER 2

NATURE AND STRUCTURE OF VIRUSES

Since the principle of most of the laboratory methods and tests for viral diagnoses are actually based on the general or specific characteristics or properties of the viruses, it will be appropriate to understand the basic structure of viruses.

A complete virus particle is called virion. The virion contains the nucleic acid which can either be ribonucleic acid (RNA) or deoxyribonucleic acid (DNA). The nucleic acid contains all the genetic information of the virus. The nucleic acid is surrounded by an outer protective coat, the capsid. The combination of the nucleic acid and the capsid is referred to as the nucleocapsid. The capsid (morphological subunit) is made up of capsomeres which are the structural units of the virion. The capsomeres are the building block of the virus during virus assembly and maturation. The capsid is made of proteins which are encoded by the viral genome. These viral proteins form the morphological subunit of the virus and most of the time also serve as important antigenic distinctions for differentiating the virus from other group of viruses. This is an important diagnostic property. The proteins associated with the viral nucleic acid form what is known as nucleo- proteins. Since the nucleoproteins are specific and peculiar to species, groups and families, they often serve as markers for the identification of these virus and directly or indirectly of recognizing such viruses as the agents of diseases they cause. The principle of such tests for the recognition is therefore related to the structure, or the function being performed by such structure.

Viruses, especially the RNA viruses, during the process of replicating in their host, may envelop themselves with the cell membrane surrounding the infected cell or with the inner nuclear membrane during budding. Such viruses are referred to as enveloped viruses. The viral envelop is a lipid bilayer which is studded with proteins or glycoproteins encoded by the viral and infected host cell genome, the lipid membrane and the carbohydrates which are donated by the host genome. The envelop proteins are called glycoproteins. Apart from the function of protecting the virus from enzyme digestions, they also function as receptor molecules. The viral glycoproteins bind specific cellular receptor molecules thereby making the latter susceptible to infection by the virus.The glycoproteins with their receptor molecules, allow host cell to recognis and bind these virions resulting in their uptake. Following virus –cell binding, the virus penetrates the host cell. Most of the enveloped viruses use their envelope glycoproteins to specifically bind to host cells and facilitate fusion and entry. Envelope glycoproteins are very important in the diagnosis and recognition of viral diseases. Since they bear the receptor molecules, and are the first part of contact of the host with the virion, and since they also bear all the virus-encoded glycoproteins, the host immune reaction if first directed against these proteins. It is along this principle that tests directed against these glycoproteins and/or their products are derived for the recognition.

Some viruses, especially Influenza and Measles have on their envelopes, projections in form of filaments and peplomers. These projections contain virus-encoded proteins like haemagglutinins and neuranmidase, or other forms of proteins which distinguish each virus types from the other. The principle of detecting some of these proteins or products of their functions serve as very useful diagnostic tests for identifying the viruses and their effects.

Nucleic Acid Composition	Virus Family	Genome Structure	Diameter (nm)	Nucleocapsid Symmetry	Envelope	Viral Assembly Site	Family Representative
RNA	Picorna-viridae	SS	25-30	Icosahedral	N	C	Enterovirus, Rhinovirus
	Orthomyxo-viridae	SS	80-120	Helical	E	C	Influenza virus Parainfluenza
	Paramyxo-viridae	SS	150-300	Helical	E	C	Mumps Measles
	Filoviridae	SS	50-80	Helical	E	C	Ebola, Marburg
	Flaviviridae	SS	30-50	Iosahedral	E	C	Yellow Fever, Dengue, West Nile, HCV
	Reoviridae	DS	70-80	Icosahedral	N	C	Reovirus Rotavirus
	Retroviridae	SS	100-120	Icosahedral	E	C	HIV-1 HTLV-1
	Rhabdo-viridae	SS	60-180	Helical	E	C	Rabies

DNA	Herpes-viridae	DS	150-300	Icosahedral	E	Nu	HSV1,2 CMV, VZV, EBV, HHV-6
	Adeno-viridae	DS	70-80	Icosahedral	N	Nu	Adenovirus
	Polyoma-viridae	DS	45-55	Icosahedral	N	Nu	HPV,JC,BK
	Papilloma-viridae	DS	50-55		N	Nu	CIN
	Poxviridae	DS	230-300	Complex	N	Nu	Vaccinia
	Parvoviridae	SS	18-20	Icosahedral	N	Nu	B19

N=Non-enveloped
E=Enveloped
C=Cytoplasm
Nu=Nucleus

Table 2.1. Classification and Nature of some Important Viral Families

Further Reading
1. Crick FHC and Watson J.D. "Structure of small Viruses." *Nature* 177: 473 1956.
2. Elsevier Science and Technology Books, New York, 1974.
3. Fenner F., Mims C., Sambrook J. and McAusland B. *The Biology of Animal Viruses.*
4. Raph R.K. *Double Stranded Viral RNA. Adv Virus Research* 15: 61, 1969.
5. Steere RL, Schaffer FL. *The Structure of Crystals of Purified Maloney Poliovirus* Acta *Biochem Biophys* 195: 28: 241.
6. Temin H.M and Batimore D. *"RNA directed DNA Synthesis and RNA Tumor Viruses." Adv Virus Res.* 17: 129: 1972.

CHAPTER 3

QUALITY ASSURANCE IN THE VIROLOGY LABORATORY

With the central role that laboratories are playing in the treatment and management of patients, coupled with the large amount of samples and the urgency to release diagnostic test results for the treatment of patients, the impact of any laboratory error will be enormous. Adequate and sufficient arrangement must be put in place for the provision of reliable and accurate test result. Therefore, quality assurance in the virology laboratory is essential for the monitoring and improvement of all the activities in the laboratory. Quality assurance extends beyond the laboratory internal process but includes patient preparation, sampling, testing, reporting, notification and test interpretation all of which must be subjected to scrutiny that are guided by standardised regulations by regulatory bodies. There are different levels of regulatory bodies that regulate the activities of laboratories in Nigeria.

The purpose of these bodies is to improve the qualities of the laboratory, to ensure that accurate and reliable results are achieved. Accreditation of such laboratories by the regulatory bodies are done annually during which time, personnel qualifications, responsibility and competency assessments, are undertaken. An important aspect of the quality assurance is the annual proficiency testing which measures the ability of the laboratory to maintain standard set by regulatory body. It is also the responsibility of the regulatory body to make sure that standard operating procedure (SOP) are maintained by the laboratory. As part of the quality assurance, the laboratory must provide a means of checking the verification and validation of tests, monitor the condition of reagents, provide evidence of equipment quality control and preoperative maintenance.

Quality Control

A very important component of the quality assurance in the laboratory is the daily monitoring of equipment, reagents, and environmental conditions. Procedures and results must be documented and displayed openly in the laboratory and any corrected action must be taken immediately. The temperature of all heat-related equipments must be checked and recorded daily. The level of the liquid nitrogen in the nitrogen tanks and humidity of the incubators must be checked. All these result must be within the standard values required. Reagent and reagent bottles must be checked for correct labelling, concentration and purity. Equally important is the date of preparation and expiration of reagents, such as buffers, media and other related reagents like antibiotics and other chemicals

Cell Culture Quality Control

The cell culture is a very important component of the virology laboratory The cell culture quality control as practised in the polio laboratory is a very good example of cell quality control. This can be applied to any other cell culture laboratory. Cell culture records must show the type of cells, the number of passages, source of cells and date received in the laboratory and finally the type of media used. The number of passages in the laboratory of receipt is the number of passages from the source plus 1. On receipt of cells, they are allowed to rest in the incubator for 24 hours in the original medium after which they are sub-cultured into new flasks. In case the cells are not confluent on arrival, the volume of the shipping medium should be reduced to $1/10^{th}$ of the original volume. This is to increase the oxygen tension inside the flask. Cells can be stored away after the second passage. Cells are stored when they are in active growth. Cells are passaged fifteen times before they are discarded. Within these fifteen passages, cells sensitivity must be carried out three times preferably on receipt and on the seventh and fifteenth passages.

Part of the cell culture quality control includes checking for mycoplasma contamination and type of cytopathic effect. Culture media and other reagents must be checked for identity, pH, growth promotion and absence of toxicity. The water in the tissue culture laboratory must be tissue-culture grade, free from pyrogens and bacteria. Primary cell lines must be checked for adventitious agents. Finally, as part of the quality control, working tables and benches must be well disinfected with 10% sodium hypochlorite and all work must be done in a class II bio-safety cabinet with HEPA filter.

Laboratory Manual

The laboratory manual is an essential tool in the laboratory. The manual is a detailed documentation of stepwise procedures of tasks performed and which are guided by and are within the requirement of the regulating body. The laboratory manual must give the title of each task and the test principle involved. Also the laboratory manual explains procedure for sample collection, transportation and storage. Other important aspects of the quality assurance that must be in the laboratory manual include information on reagent standard and control, sources of supplier, instrument calibration and maintenance, quality control frequency and acceptable limits, test steps, calculations, expected values, limitation of methods, methods of validation, implementation and update dates on trouble shooting and corrective measures taken. All these results must be within the recommended standard values. The laboratory procedure must be reviewed and approved by the Director or Head of the laboratory and updated if necessary.

Staff

All the staff in the virology laboratory must be professionally qualified to work in the laboratory. In Nigeria, any holder of the OND or HND with specialisation in microbiology or virology may be qualified as a technical staff in the virology laboratory. Specific special areas may however require further training. University degrees holders in any of the life sciences, medical sciences are qualified as scientific officers. However, the most important factor is that the staff must be proficient, trainable and experienced.

Safety in the Laboratory

Safety is paramount in the laboratory. Viruses are infectious agents. There have been many reported cases in which laboratorians died of viral infections contacted during disease investigations. Evaluation of safety, therefore, constitutes one of the important quality assurance issues considered during laboratory accreditation and inspection by the regulatory body.

The goals of laboratory safety programme are to provide a place to work with little or no risk. Routine procedures should be such as to minimise laboratory accidents while equipment constitute no source of danger. Hazards materials must be restricted and staff should be well trained on the handling of such hazardous materials.

Four categories of laboratory hazards are recognised: physical, microbiological, chemical and radiological.

Infection through aerosol, contamination of skin, eyes, mucous membrane, accidental self puncture and ingestion are all but possible in the virology laboratory. Infection can occur during handling of specimens and culture of viruses. Laboratorians have been infected while handling cells from animal origin because of endogenous agents contained in such cells. Laboratorians should treat all clinical materials coming into the laboratory as potentially dangerous and therefore adhere to the safety regulations.

Biosafety Levels

The biosafety levels are the different required precautionary means, equipment and materials for handling the various infectious viruses depending on the virulence, infectivity pathogenesis and mode of spread of these viruses

The Centers for Disease Control and Prevention (CDC) and the National Institute of Health (NIH) have developed guidelines for handling infectious agents.

Four biosafety levels with accompanying facilities, equipment and practices are recognised. (Table 3.1). These levels are proportional to the severity of diseases associated with the infectious agents and the capacity for transmission via the aerosol.

Risk	Biosafety level	Examples of Laboratories	Laboratory Practices	Safety Equipments
1	Biosafety Level 1	Basic Teaching	Good microbiological technique	None. Open bench work
2	Biosafety Level 2	Primary health services, diagnostic, teaching and public health	Protective clothing, bioharzar signs	Open bench, Bio-safety cabinet
3	Containment-Biosafety Level 3	Special Diagnostic	As level 2 plus special clothing, controlled access, directional air-flow	Biosafety Cabinet and/or other primary containment
4	Maximum containment Level 4	Dangerous pathogen Unit	As level 3 plus airlock entry, shower exit, special waste disposal	Class III Biosafety Cabinet or positive pressure suits, double ended autoclave, filtered air

Table-3.1 Biosafety Levels

Specific safety rules for personnel must be followed. What are these safety rules:

(a) The laboratory personnel must wear the appropriate personnel protective equipment (PPE) when working in the virology laboratory. These PPE include lab coats, gloves safety glasses and mouth gag if applicable.

(b) All vials containing virus must be well capped.

(c) Aerosol generating activities like centrifugation, sonication, blending, forceful expulsion of contents from needle and syringes and vacuutainer tubes must be carefully handled with the containment equipment.

(d) Mouth pipetting is strictly forbidden.

(e) Contaminated pipette must never be put on the surface of work bench.

(f) Virus containing -fluids must never be sent down the sink.

(g) Eating, drinking and smoking are strictly prohibited in the laboratory.

(h) Bench tops and biosafety cabinet tops should be thoroughly disinfected after each day.

(i) At the end of each day or task, gloves and lab coats should be removed and hands washed with soap and disinfectant.

(j) Continuous training of staff on safety procedure must be in place.

(k) Laboratorians working with specific viruses should be immunised against these viruses and against those viruses suspected to be present in those samples frequently processed by the laboratorians, if vaccines are available.

Further Reading
WHO Laboratory Biosafety Manual (2nd ed) World Health Organisation Geneva 1993.

CHAPTER 4

CLINICAL SPECIMENS – THEIR COLLECTION, TRANSPORT AND PROCESSING

Collection

Viruses can only be successfully isolated from clinical specimens when such specimens are collected at the right time and handled appropriately. Specimens should be collected at such a time when the virus is available in the specimen in high amount, i.e. when the titre is high. This period, most of the time, corresponds to the acute phase of the disease, which for most viral diseases fall within three days after onset of clinical manifestation. Usually, any time longer than that, antibodies that are likely to neutralize out the virus begin to appear. Specimens should be correctly labelled, showing patient's name, age and sex, date of collection, date of onset, clinical symptoms and presumptive diagnosis. Information on specimens will most likely lead the laboratory personnel to the choice of the type and sensitivity of the test to use. Specimens for virus isolation should be transported to the laboratory immediately in reverse cold chain i.e. in a well packed cold box with cold ice-packs. (Fig.4 1). For example, for polio isolation, samples collected in the field must reach the laboratory within 72 hours after collection. Specimen may be kept at – 70°C if it would be impossible to get it to the laboratory within three days.

Type of Specimen

The selection of the right specimen is dictated by the clinical symptoms, the presumptive diagnosis and the virus suspected. Many viruses can give the same clinical symptoms while a virus may also give several clinical syndromes. It is therefore important that the appropriate specimens are collected. From a patient showing central nervous system involvement suspected to be enterovirus, cerebro-spinal fluids (CSF), throat and rectal swabs and stools may be collected. A CNS involvement with parotitis where mump is suspected, urine and CSF can be collected. The best specimen for measles will be blood collected within threes days after the appearance of rash or urine which could still be collected fourteen days after onset of clinical symptoms. (Table 4.1)

Virus isolation may not always be possible for most of the diseases. In such cases, convalescent sera for serology will be a better choice. With the availability of PCR in most laboratories today, specimens for virus isolation can also be used for nucleic acid amplification of the viral nucleic acid.

Specimens should be collected in the right amount. Stool for polio virus isolation should be about five grams, i.e. the size of the thumb. Usually, between five to ten milliliters of blood are adequate for serology and viral studies. Swabs and tissues should be collected in viral transport medium made up of Balanced Salt Solution (BSS) supplemented with 0.5% gelatin, 2% fetal calf serum (FCS) or bovine serum albumin in the absence of FCS. Antibiotics and fungicides must be added to prevent bacterial and fungal growth while in transit. Some commercial virus transport media (VTM) are available in the market.

Specimen Transportation

In this time of heightened international security, transportation of specimens across international borders is posing a great challenge. Most airlines are rejecting specimens they classify as hazardous or dangerous, while those that accept them need security permits to cover their operation. This underscores the need to carefully package these specimens to avoid leakage or contact with outside while maintaining the cold-chain.

A typical WHO approved container for the transportation of poliovirus specimens which could either be stool or virus isolate between laboratory consists of isothermal packaging box with an inner specimen container and ice-packs is shown in Fig 4.1

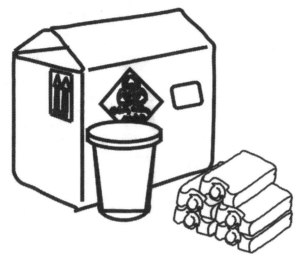

Fig. 4.1 Cold Box for the transportation of infectious virus materials

Clinical Condition	Viruses Suspected	Samples for Collection	Possible Laboratory Test
Lower Respiratory Tract Infection	Influenza A, B, Adenoviruses, RSV	Bronchoaveolar lavage, nasal swab, lung biopsy,	Virus isolation in culture, PCR, IF
Upper Respiratory Tract Infection	Rhinovirus , RSV, Adenovirus, Parainfluenza, Influenza A,B	Nasal wash, Nasal swab, Nasopharyngeal swab, Throat swab.	Virus isolation in culture,IF, PCR
Myocarditis, Pericarditis	Enterovirus	Stool, Blood, endocardial biopsy, throat swab	Virus isolation in TC, PCR
	Influenza	Throat swab, endocardial biopsy,	Virus isolation in TC, PCR
	CMV	Throat swab, urine, endocardial biopsy	Virus isolation in TC, PCR
Gastroenteritis	Rotavirus Norovirus(Nor walk Agent)	Stool Stool, serum	EM, IEM, ELISA, PCR
	Adenovirus, CMV	Stool, Colon biopsy	EM, ELISA,Virus isolation in TC. Virus isolation in TC
	Enterovirus	Stool.	
Cutaneous and mucous membrane Infections	HSV, VZV, Vaccinia	Lesion swab,	Virus isolation in TC, Serology,PCR

(Vesicular or exanthematous)	Measles	Blood, Urine, Serum	Virus isolation in TC, Serology(ELISA, IF), PCR
	Enteroviruses	Throat swab, Stool	Virus isolation in TC, Serology Serology(IgM ELISA, HI) Virus Isolation in TC
	Rubella	Serum, CSF,Throat swab, Nasopharygeal secretion	Virus Isolation in TC, PCR, Serology
Central Nervous System Infections			
Acute Flaccid Paralysis	Enteroviruses	Stool,CSF, Throat swab	Virus Isolation in TC, PCR,Serology
Encephalitis	HSV,VZV,	CSF, Brain biopsy	Virus isolation in TC,PCR,Serology
Meningitis	Adenovirus, Mumps virus, Influenza ,	CSF,Throat swab,Urine,	Serology (ELISA,IF,FAMA. Virus Isolation in TC
	HIV	Serum,CSF, Blood	Virus Isolation in TC
	Enterovirus	CSF, Stool,Throat swab	ELISA,Virus isolation in TC, PCR
	HSV	CSF, Stool,Throat swab	Virus Isolation in TC
	Mumps	CSF,Urine, Serum	Virus Isolation in TC Serology, PCR Virus Isolation in TC, Serology, PCR
AIDS	HIV-1, HIV-2	Plasma, Serum, Blood	ELISA, Westernblot, PCR(Viral Load)

Hepatitis	Hepatitis A, B, C, D, E	Serum	Serology(ELISA, IF, RIA),
		Liver tissue	
	CMV,HSV, Adenovirus EBV	Serum	Virus Isolation in TC Serology

TC=Tissue Culture

PCR=Polymerase Chain Reaction

EM=Electron microscopy

IEM=Immune electron microscopy

IF=Immunoflourescent

ELISA=Enzyme Linked Immunosorbent Assay

HI=Heamagglunitation Inhibition

FAMA=fluorescent antibody membrane assay

RIA=Radioimmunoassay

CSF=Cerebrospinal Fluid

Table 4.1 Specimens for diagnosis of viral infections and diseases

SPECIMEN	METHODS OF COLLECTION
Throat Swab	Vigorously but carefully scrub the posterior pharynx and tonsils. Immediately place the swab inside the VTM.
Nasal Swab	Scrub and rotate swab gently in the two nostrils to obtain enough secretion and epithelia if possible.
Nasopharyngeal Aspirate	Insert the catheter into posterior nasopharyx. Aspirate mucus into a mucus trap and with VTM, PBS or saline, wash the mucus through the suction catheter and into trap.
Nasopharyngeal Swab	Gently insert flexible swab into the nasopharyx. Rotate gently. Remove and place inside the VTM.
Bronchoalveolar Lavage	Wedge the bronchoscope into subsegmental bronchus . Insert four 50 ml boluses of sterile saline into the suction port with immediate return suction after the insertion of each sample. Submit 5-10ml for viral studies.
	With a 13 gauge needle, collect about 2 ml into a sterile vial.

Table 4.2 Specimen Collection

Specimen Processing

The method used for processing specimens for virus isolation will depend on the nature of specimens. However, the most important fact is that such method must be such as to give the best chance of virus recovery.

Stools for poliovirus and other enteroviruses are processed by chloroform treatment (Fig.4. 2). About 3-5gms of stool is placed in a 50ml centrifuge tube and 10ml of phosphate buffered saline (PBS) is added. Sterile glass beads are added. One ml of laboratory grade chloroform ($CHCl_3$) is layered over the PBS. The tube with content is then shaken manually or mechanically by a shaker for 10 minutes. The tube can now be spun in a cold centrifuge at 3000 rpm for 10 minutes. The chloroform destroys all the organic materials as well as bacteria, fungi, parasites and other chloroform sensitive viruses present in the stool with no adverse effect on the three polio types and the other enteroviruses. The liquid layer containing the virus is carefully removed and dispensed in cryovals in 0.5-1ml aliquots. The processed specimen can either be inoculated immediately into a sensitive cell line or stored away at -20^0C or -40^0C.

Stool Processing

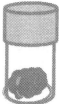

Stool Sample
Organic material
Bacteria
Fungi
Parasites
Polio Sabin 1-3
Polio Wild 1-3
Other enteros
Other viruses

Fig 4.2. Treatment of stool for poliovirus and other enterovirus isolation. (*Adapted with permission from WHO Polio Manual, 2nd ed. WHO Geneva 2004)*

For other viruses, swabs are broken into tubes containing 2ml of VTM. The content of the swab will flow into the transport medium. This can be gently vortexed and inoculated in 0.1.-0.2ml amounts into the appropriate cell culture.

Urine specimen must be diluted out 1:2 to reduce cell toxicity before inoculation. It may also be necessary to adjust the pH to slightly neutral or basic pH (7.0-7.4). This can be done with 7.5% 1N sodium bicarbonate.

Bronchoalveolar lavage must be centrifuged at about 3000 rpm for 20 minutes and resuspended in about 5mls of PBS before inoculation. Sputum must be broken down in VTM with glass beads. About 4mls of VTM is enough depending on the volume and nature of the sputum. The container can be vortexed and supernatant inoculated directly into cell culture.

Whole tissues or organs and autopsy or biopsy tissues are usually processed by homogenisation and grinding for virus release. Home or ordinary kitchen homogenisers or blenders can be used provided it is only for laboratory use only. Hard tissues will need to be minced with sterile scissors in medium without serum or in PBS to which 0.25% trypsin is added. The minced tissue can be transferred into a sterile centrifuge tube containing growth medium. The tube is centrifuged at 3000 rmp for 15 minutes and cells resuspended in VTM to give a final concentration of 20% v/v. Soft tissues can be homogenised by grinding or passing through sterile syringes.

Separation of white blood cells from whole blood

Cell associated viruses like measles and CMV are easily isolated from the blood leukocyte fractions. This includes the lymphocytes, mononuclear and polymorphonuclear cells.

Leukocytes fractions can be separated from fresh whole blood using one of two methods described below:

1 Ficoll – Hypaque

The F-H method yields lymphocytes and monocytes.

(a) Fresh blood is collected in anticoagulant which can either be heparin or Alservers solution usually between 0.2 to 0.5-ml of anticoagulant in 5-10ml of fresh blood.

(b) Mix equal volume of whole blood with cold PBS.

(c) Gently overlay Ficoll-Hypaque with the diluted whole blood in the ratio of 3 volumes of whole blood to 1 volume of F-H, being careful not to mix the two interphases.

(d) Centrifuge at 3500 rpm (400xg) for 30 minutes at room temperature.

(e) Remove the top plasma and platelet layer, again being careful not to mix the interphase together.

(f) With the aid of sterile pipette, gently aspirate the mononuclear layer into another centrifuge tube and add about 5ml of serum free medium.

(g) Centrifuge at 900xg for 10 minutes. Discard the supernatant.

(h) Repeat the washing by adding about 10mls of serum free medium and centrifuge at the same speed.

(i) Add about 2ml of VTM to the leucocyte pellets. The leucocytes can be inoculated into susceptible cells at this point. They can also be co-cultured with the cells.

2. Dextran Separation Method

This method is used for those viruses where combined leucocyte fractions i.e. mononuclear, polymorphonuclear and lymphocytes are needed for the virus isolation, e.g. CMV. This method is faster and simpler compared to the F-H method.

(a) Two parts of whole blood is mixed with one part of 6% dextran (MW 70,000) in a centrifuge tube and incubated at 37^{oC} for 30 minutes. This allows the red blood cell to settle.

(b) The leucocyte- rich supernatant is gently removed from the red blood cell sediment and transferred to another centrifuge tube containing 5-7mls of serum free medium.

(c) The mixture is then centrifuged at 900 x g for 10 minutes while the supernatant is discarded.

(d) The washing is continued, this time, adding 5-7ml of serum free medium. At this point, the leucocytes may still be containing some erythrocytes. This can be lysed off by quickly adding sterile distilled water with shaking for 5-10 seconds.

(e) Quickly add 10ml of 2% MEM to stop the lysis. Recentrifuge at 900g for 10 minutes and resuspend in 2ml VTM. The cell is ready for inoculation.

Bone marrow can be treated like blood if it is an aspirate, but if it is a biopsy, it should be homogenised.

Virus Transport Media(VTM)

Hanks Gelatinised Balanced Salt Solution

Hanks Balanced Salt	100ml
Gelatin	0.5 g

Sterilise by autoclaving at 15 lbs/in^2 for 15 minutes. Add antibiotics to desired concentration and dispense in 2-3.5ml aliquots. This can be stored at 4°C.

Buffered Tryptose Phosphate Broth with Gelatin

Tryptose Phosphate Broth	2.9g
$Na_2HPO4.7H_2O$	2.06g
$NaH_2PO_4.H_2O$	0.08g
Gelatin	0.50g
Phenol Red(0.5%)	0.40ml
Distilled Water	100.00ml

Sterilise by autoclaving at 15lbs for 15 minutes. Add antibiotics. Store as above.

Infusion Broth

Veal Infusion Broth	2.5g
Phenol Red	0.4ml
Distilled Water	100.00ml

Sterilise by autoclaving as above. Add 0.5 g of bovine serum albumin after cooling. Sterilise by filtration through 0.45 um Millipore filter. Add antibiotics and fungizones before use. Store as above.

Further Reading

Dulbecco, R. and Ginsberg H.S. *Virology 3rd ed.* Haperstown Md: Harper & Row Inc. 1980

Fenner F.O. and White D.O. *Medical Virology 3rd ed.* New York: Academic Press 1976.

Hsiung G.D. ed. *Recent Advances in Clinical Virology.* New Yolk. Praeger 1980

Lennette EH, Schmidt NJ, eds (1979). *Diagnostic procedures for viral, rickettsial and chlamydial infections,* 5th ed. Washington, DC, American Public Health Association.

WHO Polio Laboratory Manual 4th ed Immunisation, Vaccines and Biologicals. World Health Organisation, Geneva, Switzerland 2004.

PART II

DIAGNOSTIC METHODS FOR ISOLATING AND IDENTIFYING VIRUSES

CHAPTER 5

Virus Isolation

One of the major characteristics that differentiate viruses from other microorganisms is their inability to grow in non-living tissues but only in susceptible living tissues. Virus isolation is very important and basic for any study on the nature, morphology and properties of a virus. Virus isolation forms the basis of identification and detection of the virus. It is the most sensitive and accurate method of identification and diagnosis of viral infection and is regarded as the gold standard for virus identification, classification and diagnosis. The introduction of tissue culture into virology has facilitated the study of viruses tremendously and has also led to the development of many control and diagnostic materials such as vaccines and other biological products.

While cell culture remains the most commonly used method for virus isolation because of some perceived advantages, embryonated eggs, small and large animals, are also good sources for virus isolation.

Virus Isolation in Cell Culture
Cell culture is the process by which prokaryotic, eukaryotic or plant cells are grown under controlled conditions. The discovery that polio virus would grow in cells of non-neural origin opened the way for the use of cell culture for isolation of many viruses. Two types of cell lines

are usually available – the established cell line and the primary cell line. At present, many different cells lines are available for isolation of various viruses.(Table 5.1) Although most of these cells are available from sources like American Type Culture Collection (ATCC) and other sources, many laboratories can actually prepare cells in their primary form. Homologous primary cell lines are usually more sensitive for primary isolation of viruses. Cells can be grown in cell culture tubes, flasks and bottles, using the appropriate cell culture media. Because of the presence of different surface receptors on the cells, not all viruses will grow in the same cell line, and not all cell lines will permit the growth of a particular virus. Cells that permit the growth of a particular virus is referred to as susceptible. Before inoculating a suspension in to the cell, the cell must be allowed to form a confluent monolayer. This can be achieved by growing the cell in the appropriate medium in the presence of growth medium, which is usually supplemented with 10% fetal calf serum (FCS). Confluent monolayer can be inoculated with the inoculum for virus isolation as follows:

Bring out the cells to be inoculated from the incubator onto the cleaned surface of the biosafety cabinet.

Pour off the medium and rinse with warm PBS(37°C) to remove any coating serum that may prevent virus attachment.

With a sterile pipette, inoculate between 0.1-0.2 ml of your inoculum. The volume of the inoculum can be increased depending on the size of the monolayer of cell.

Incubate at the appropriate temperature (usually 35-37°C) for one hour for virus adsorbtion, rocking the cell culture vessels every 15 minutes to prevent dehydration.

Add the appropriate volume of maintenance medium containing 2% FCS.

Label the inoculated material (tube, flask or bottle) indicating date of inoculation and material inoculated.

Incubate at the appropriate temperature (usually 35-37°C) and check daily for cytopathic effect (CPE) for seven days. Medium may have to be changed the third day post inoculation (pi) if there is no evidence of viral effect.

If there is no CPE, a second passage is done and observed for another 7 days. Cells showing CPE during the period of incubation are harvested for virus identification and further study. If there is no CPE after the second passage, the specimen is regarded as negative for the suspected virus.

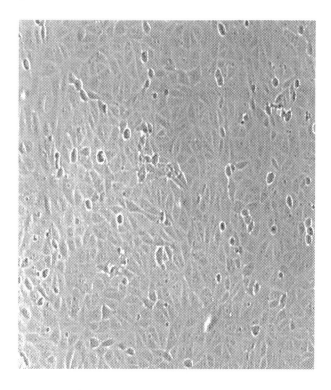

Fig.5.1. Uninfected Vero Cell Line.

The Vero cell is of the African green monkey origin and is found virtually in all virology laboratories where tissue cultures are used. It is permissive to a lot of viruses both for primary and secondary isolation

For viruses like influenza that may not show possible CPE, presence of virus may be detected by heamadsorbtion.
Isolated viruses can be identified by the type of CPE (cell rounding, foamy, syncytia, giant multinucleated cells etc.) Final identification must, however, be done by serological tests such as neutralisation test using monoclonal antibodies or known positive sera to the virus suspected. Isolates can also be identified by haemagglutination inhibition test and complement fixation test (see procedures under specific test).

Cell Culture	Name	Origin	Virus Susceptibility
Primary	HEK	Human Embryo Kidney	Adenovirus, HSV, Enteroviruses Mumps Measles
	MK	Monkey Kidney	Enteroviruses, Rhinoviruses, Reoviruses, Influenza virus, Parainfluenza virus, Mumps
	RK	Rabbit Kidney	HSV
	CEF	Chicken Embryo Fibroblast	Influenza, NDV,
	GPE	(Guinea pig embryo	HSV, Coxsackie A
Diploid Cell Line	WI-38 MRC -5 HDF	Human diploid fibroblast(Lung	CMV, VZV,HSV,RSV, Mumps, Enteroviruses.

Transformed/ Est-ablished	Vero	African Green Monkey	A variety of viruses
	Hep-2	Human Larynx Carcinoma	RSV, Adeno, HSV, Polio, Coxsackie B, Rhinoviruses
	B95-8, B95a	EBV Transformed Marmoset	Measles
	RD	Human Rhabdomyosarcoma	Polio, Non-polio enteroviruses
	L20B	Mouse L cell(CD155 transgenic)	Poliovirus, Certain Adeno.
	HeLa	Human Cervix Carcinoma	Rhino, Adeno, RSV, HSV.
	BHK-21	Baby Hamster Kidney	Rubella, Vaccinia, Arbovirus
	RK-13	Rabbit Kidney	Rubella

Table 5.1 Some Common Cell Lines for Virus Isolation.

Virus Isolation in Mice

The mouse is another good host for virus isolation. Most viruses will grow in mice when inoculated intra-cerebrally into newborn mice. Some groups of Coxsackie viruses and the Flaviviruses are easily isolated in mice. The Swiss white albino mouse is commonly found in most virological laboratories. The younger the animal, the more susceptible. Animals like rabbit, guinea pigs and hamsters may be inoculated with viruses but more for antibody production rather than for virus isolation. For intracerebral inoculation, between 0.01-0.02 ml of inoculum is inoculated into the brain between the visible veins using 28 inch gauge needle.

For intraperitoneal inoculation between 0.03-0.05ml inoculum is deposited in the peritoneum, using a 25 inch gauge needle.

Inoculated mice must be checked daily for death or paralysis. The death occurring within 12-24 hours post inoculation is regarded as non-specific virus death. The brain of dead mice or those showing paralysis can be harvested and made into a 10% suspension for further inoculation or virus study.

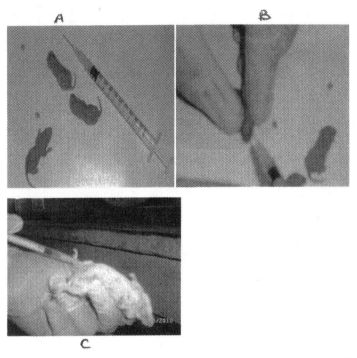

Fig. 5.2. Mice inoculation with virus suspension: (A) One day-old white albino mice (B) Intracerebral inoculation (C) Intraperitoneal inoculation

Isolation in embryonated chicken

Fertile embryonated eggs provide another good system for virus isolation because they prove very sensitive to viruses like influenza and mumps viruses. The best age for inoculation is 10-12 day old. Before inoculation, the part of the egg to deposit the inoculum must be decided, whether in the chorio allantoic membrane, (CAM) amniontic sac, or the yolk sac depending on the type of virus. This will depend on the virus being suspected.

Embryonated eggs must be candled before inoculation to determine the viability of the embryo, identify the locations for inoculation, and locate the arteries and veins.

For amniotic and allantoic cavity inoculation, the following steps can be taken:

Use embryonaed eggs between the ages of 7-8 days for mumps virus and 10-13 for influenza virus.

Candle the eggs, disinfect the air sac with iodine and puncture with egg puncher.

Mark the position for your inoculation.

Still under the candler, inoculate between 0.1 – 0.2 ml of your inoculum into the amnioitic sac or allantoic cavity using a 23" gauge needle.

Seal the hole on the egg shell with paraffin wax.

Incubate the inoculated eggs at 35-37°C. Eggs must be placed in upright position with the air sac up.

Candle the eggs daily. Usually any egg that dies within the first 24 hours is regarded as non-specific death and should be discarded.

Dead eggs should be removed and kept refrigerated at 4°C ready for harvest.

Harvest the amniotic or allantoic fluid.

Embryonated eggs can be harvested by cutting open the air-sac. The egg and the whitish chorioallantoic membranes are carefully removed using capillary pipette or syringe. The allantoic or amniotic fluids are carefully aspirated into a sterile container.

These fluids are ready for whatever further test that may be required for identification of the virus.

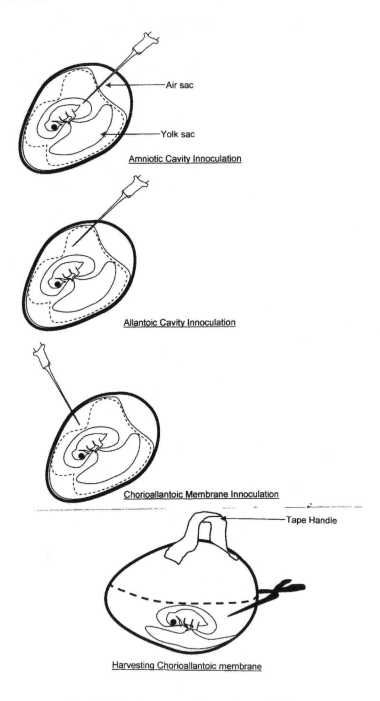

Fig 5.3 Embryonated eggs inoculation.

Chorioallantoic membrane route

The choroiallantoic membrane route is a bit more difficult and delicate than the previous two. It is commonly used for those viruses that form pocks.

Observing the 9-12 old eggs under the candler, carefully mark areas free from the arteries and veins.

Make two slits, one on the site of inoculation and the second on the air-sac.

Carefully remove the slits, exposing the white chorioallantoic membrane. Puncture the air-sac and with a sterile pipette with bulb, create a suction in the air-sac.

Inoculate about 0.05ml of the inoculum into the collapsed CAM. Seal the slit and the air sac with paraffin wax or tape, and incubate egg at 35-37°C.

Candle the eggs daily. Dead eggs can be kept away at 4°C till ready for harvest. Carefully remove the CAM and observe for pocks.

Inoculation of embryonated egg blood vessels

This method is rarely used. It is used for those viruses which will neither grow in any of the other routes. Example of such virus is the Bluetongue virus.

CHAPTER 6

Cell Culture in Virology

Cell culture techniques became very prominent in virology laboratory and research in the 1940s and 1950s and have currently provided the most widely used and most powerful hosts for cultivation and assay of viruses.

Most viruses can be isolated in culture, which facilitated the study of their structure, nature, physical and chemical properties, identification and typing. The introduction of tissue culture also led to the production of control agents like vaccines.

In an ideal virology laboratory, a combination of different types of cells should be available at any time. These should include primary monkey kidney cells, human diploid cell, or human cells lines having heteroploid markers. This is to allow for a broad spectrum possibility of isolating viruses from clinical samples as they are brought for virus isolation and identification.

There are three types of culture –
(i)   organ culture,
(ii)   primary explant culture (tissue culture) and
(iii)   cell culture.

Organ culture retains the original three-dimensional architecture of the tissue. The primary explant culture is derived by mincing pieces of tissue in liquid medium from which the individual cells continue to grow without having to disintegrate. In cell culture, the tissue is disintegrated into the individual cells before culturing, using a chelating agent such as trypsin.

Cell culture can be categorised into three depending on the length of time they could remain in culture. These are primary cell culture, cell strain and cell line. Each of these cell cultures possesses its own characteristics and viruses behave differently on these cultures. Primary cell lines are often more sensitive for primary isolation of viruses.

Primary cell lines are those obtained from their original tissue and which have not been subcultured. These cells have limited life-span and cannot continue to grow indefinitely. Primary cell lines can be grown from different species of animals – small, large, newborn animals, embryos of human or monkey origin, rodents, rats, mice, embryonated eggs, and birds.

Primary cell lines can be subcultured many times but not indefinitely. During the period between the first culture and the time they essentially die out (crisis or senescence) the cells are referred to as cell strain.

Cell strains can become transformed such that they become immortalised. Immortalisation can occur during continuous passage of the cell strains or by use of chemical mutagen and infection with tumorigenic viruses. Immortalised cell cultures are called cell-lines (continuous, established cell lines).

Continuous passage of cultured cells may give rise to specific variants which can lead to a change in the character of such cell line, for example, change in sensitivity of cell to virus. It is therefore advisable that to retain the vital characteristics of cells in the virology laboratory, cells should be banked at lower passage from which stocks are obtained at given period. Usually cell should be discarded after the fifteenth passage. (See Table 5.1)

Primary cell culture is widely acknowledged as the best cell culture systems available since they support the widest range of viruses. However, reliable supply is often difficult to obtain. Continuous cells are the most easy to handle but the range of viruses supported is often limited.

Media for growth of cells in culture

Medium is by far the most important single factor in culturing cells and tissues. The choice of which medium to use and what supplement to add is strongly influenced by the nature and type of cell to be grown. The function of the medium is to provide the enabling environment and physical condition of the growth of the cells and its survival. This physical condition includes the pH, osmotic pressure, temperature, e.t.c. Medium also provides the complex chemical substances required by the tissue which it cannot synthesise on is own.

There are two types of cell culture media –Natural media and Artificial or Defined media. Examples of natural media are serum, plasma and tissue extracts while examples of defined media are the commercially available and analytically defined media such as E199, MEM, DMEM, RPMI-1640 etc.

Each medium has its own balanced salt solution (BSS). The most commonly available are the Hanks BSS and Earle's BSS. Formulated media contains proteins, amino acid, hormones, serum at their optimum concentration to promote growth of some specific cell lines.

Media are categorised into growth and maintenance medium in terms of their serum contents. Growth media contain 10% of fetal calf serum (FCS) while maintenance medium contains 1-2%. Ideally, the medium should be an accurately defined mixture of chemical substances.

Serum

Serum, usually fetal calf serum (FCS) or bovine calf serum (BCS) is added to medium to stimulate growth. It interacts with virtually every other variable in the culture system. Serum serves as a source of macromolecular growth factor that is essential for multiplication of cells in culture. Serum contains a large number of different growth promoting substances in a physiologically balanced blend. One of the functions of the serum is to reduce the inhibitory effects of both contaminants and essential nutrients that are in excess. Serum macromolecule can buffer toxic mixtures by binding them and releasing them in small amounts. Serum proteins neutralise trypsin and other proteases thereby allowing the cells to overcome the damage caused by harsh subculturing. Serum provides carrier protein for water insoluble substances such as lipids.

Preparation of Primary Cell Culture

Primary cell culture can be prepared from a variety of animals – monkey, rabbit, mice, embryonated egg, cattle and sheep. The animal of choice will depend on the type of virus to be grown or isolated. The choice of specific organs will also depend on the virus. However the organ most commonly used in the virology laboratory are kidneys from embryos or fetuses, whole embryo from mice, or fertile eggs etc. Specialised cells may, however, be prepared from suitable tissues for special studies.

Preparation of primary cell culture demands a high level aseptic technique, and therefore every step to contain contamination must be maintained right from the period of preparation of instruments, equipment, supplies, media and solutions to the final stage of handling and seeding of tissues and cells.

Preferably a day or two to the time of the preparation, all instruments and supplies must have been sterilised and ready for use. Clean laboratory coats must be worn and the hands must be gloved. Preparation and handling must be done under a biological safety cabinet.

Supplies and Equipment

Surgical equipments – scissors, and forceps
Tissue culture flasks
Magnetic stirrer and bar
Sterile gauze
Funnels
Petri dishes
Centrifuge tubes 15, 30, 250ml volume

Cylinders 50, 2500, 500 and 1000ml
Pipettes 1, 2, 5, 10ml
Tissue culture plates and flasks T25, T75, T150
Haematocytometer

Media and Solutions

0.25% Trypsin-Versene
Penicillin 200μ/ml.
Streptomycin 200μ/ml.
Fungizone 50μ/ml.
Growth and maintenance media
Phosphate Buffered Saline (PBS), Hanks BSS, Trypan Blue

Preparation of Kidney Cell Culture

Kidney for the preparation of cell culture can be obtained from the animal species of choice. This will be determined by the type of virus to be isolated and the susceptility of such virus to the cell.

Open the abdomen, aseptically remove the kidneys and place them in a Petri dish containing about 10ml of Hanks Balanced Salt Solution.

Use sterile pair of scissors and forceps; remove the outer capsule from the kidney as well as any pieces of tissues and blood vessels. Cut the kidney into two half and remove the white medulla.

Transfer the kidney pieces from the dish to a conical flask. Wash twice with Hanks BSS to remove any left over blood. Add about 25ml of trypsin and allow to stand on the magnetic stirrer for 5 minutes. Discard the first digest. Add 30ml of trypsin and stir for 15 minutes. Care must however be taken not to over digest the fragile cells.

Filter the cells through layers of sterile gauze into 250 ml centrifuge tube containing 10ml of growth medium. This action stops further digestion by trypsin. Keep the filtrate refrigerated on ice. Repeat steps 3 and 4 until all the kidney cells have been trypsinised.

After all the cells have been digested, centrifuge at 750 rpm for 15minutes at 4°C. Discard the supernatant. Resuspent the cells in 10ml of growth medium and spin again.

Transfer the cell into a 15ml centrifuge tube and resuspend in 10ml of growth medium. Spin again at 750 rpm for 10 minutes. Discard the supernatant and finally resuspend the packed cells in 10ml of growth medium. Count the cells as described below.

Using a haematocytometer, count the number of cells and calculate the total number of living cells available.

Seed the container with the appropriate number of cells such that the cells will form a monolayer within 2-3 days.

The number of cells to be seeded can be easily calculated from the total number of cells counted and this will depend on the type of containers.

For 96-well plates, a cell concentration of 50-75,000 cells/ml per well, 24-well plate will require about 150-200,000 cells/ml per well, 12-well plate – 250,000 -300,000 cells/ml per well, 6-well plate may be seeded with 350,000 – 400,000 cells/ml. Culture tubes can be seeded with about 250,000 cells/ml. T25 flask – 450-500,000 cells/ml per well; T75 flask 750,000 cells/ml and T150 flask will take about 1 million cells/ml.

After the addition of cells, growth medium must be added before incubation.

Amount of growth medium

96-well plate- 0.3ml/well

24 well plate- 2ml/well

12 well plate -3ml/well

6 well plate -5ml/well

T25 – 5ml/well

T75 – 25ml/well

T150 – 50ml

The newly seeded cell may look a bit cloudy in the first 24 hours because of the different cells growing at the same time. This will also change the pH of the medium. This medium must be changed to maintenance medium two days after seeding. Examine the cells daily. A monolayer should be formed within 2-3 days. This is a primary cell line. It can be used for virus isolation or can further be sub-passaged. (Fig. 6.1).

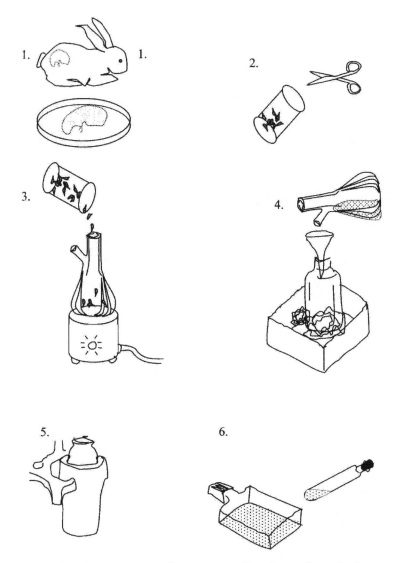

Fig. 6.1. Preparation of primary cell culture from kidney.

Chicken Embryo Fibroblast and its Preparation

The fertile egg provides a good source for the preparation of cell culture for virus isolation, especially avian viruses. Such embryonated eggs must either be specific pathogen free (SPF) or are not known to harbour intercurrent or adventitious viruses. It really does not matter whether or not the parent stocks are vaccinated against the suspected virus for isolation, the process of washing with Hanks BSS will wash away any residual maternal antibody in the embryo.

Select 9-11 day- old embryonated eggs. Candle to verify their viability. Sick embryo should not be used.

Clean the egg shell with 70% alcohol. Using a sterile pair of scissors and forceps, open up the air-sac and bring out the embryo.

Decapitate the embryo and cut off the legs. Put the torso in a sterile Petri dish containing about 10ml Hanks BSS and wash. Mince with scissors.

Transfer tissue to conical flask and wash three more times with Hanks BSS. Wash with 0.25% Trypsin for 5 minutes and discard the supernatant. Then add between 50-100 ml of 0.25% trypsin and allow to stand in a magnetic stirrer for 45 minutes, at 37°C.

Filter through sterile gauze into a centrifuge tube.

Centrifuge at 1000 rpm for 15 minutes. Pour off the supernatant to remove excess trypsin. Then wash twice with Hanks BSS at 1000 rpm for 15 minutes. Discard supernatant and finally add about 40ml of growth medium.

Refilter the suspension and centrifuge at 1000 rpm for 15 minutes. Resuspend the packed cells in cold growth medium to a final concentration of 1:10. e.g. 1ml of packed cell in 9ml of growth medium. You may count the number of cells after staining with Trypan blue.

Seed the cells as to attain confluence within 48-72 hours and incubate at 5% CO_2.

Cell Counting

To accurately determine the concentration and volume of cells to be seeded, cell counting must be done as follows:

Add 0.1ml of Trypan Blue (or any other available stain) to 0.9ml of cell suspension. This will give a 1:10 dilution. Mix by gently pipetting up and down. Avoid gas bubble.

Using a Pasteur pipette, fill the chamber of the haemocytometer, being careful not to overfill.

Count the number of live cells from the four large squares. Live cells will not be stained.

Find the average of cells and multiply by the dilution factor which in this case is 10.

Multiply by 10^4 which is the volume of the counting chamber.

Adjust cell concentration to the desired concentration. Finally multiply by the total volume of cells. This will give the number of cells per ml, (Fig. 6.2).

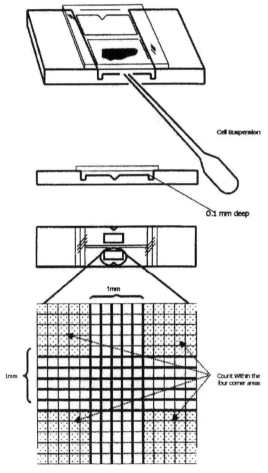

Fig. 6.2 Cell Counting (based on Freshney).
Reproduced by permission from the Polio Laboratory Manual, 4th ed. 2004.

Further Readings

Chapters 4-6

1. Clark, J. Schley. C, Irvine K, and McIntosh K. "Comparison of Cynomolgus and rhesus Monkey Kidney cells for recovery of Viruses from clinical Specimens." *J. Clin Micro* 9:554, 1979.

2. Davis BD, Dulbecco R, Eisen, HN, Givisberg HS, Wood, W.Barry and Mc Carty M. *Microbiology* 2ⁿᵈ Ed. Harper & Row Publishers Hagerstown, Mayland. 1973.

3. Hsiung G.D. "Application of Primary Cell Culture in the Study of Animal Viruses III." *Biological and Genetical Studies of Enteric Viruses of Man* (enteroviruses) Yale J Biol Med. 33: 359, 1961.

4. Howell, CL, Muller, MJ and Martin WJ. "Comparison of Rates of Viruses Isolation from Lencocyte Population Separated from Blood by Conventional and Ficoll-paque Macrodex methods." *J. Clin Micro* 10: 533, 1979.

5. Jakoby, WB and Paslan IH. *Cell Culture Methods in Enzymology.* Academic Press Inc. San Diego, California 1979. *Appl Environ Micro* 36: 480;1978.

6. Landry ML, Mayo D, and Hsiung, G.D. "Comparison of Guinea Pig Embryo Cells, Rabbit Kidney Cells and Human Embryonic Fibroblast Cell Strains for Isolation of Herpes Simplex Virus." *J. Clin. Micro* 15; 842:1982.

Schmidt NJ. HO HH, Reggs, Jl and Lenette EH. "Comparative Sensitivity of various Cell Culture Systems for Isolation of Viruses from Waste Water and Fecal Samples."

CHAPTER 7

ASSAYS FOR VIRUS IDENTIFICATION AND DIAGNOSIS

The translation of basic advances in immunochemistry, immunobiology and molecular biology into diagnostic and therapeutic procedures is the bedrock of modern clinical medicine. Various tests based on the knowledge of these disciplines are available in many laboratories today. Some of these tests have given rise to rapid detection of disease agents in the clinical sample of patients. The results of these tests are utilised by physicians in the final diagnosis and treatment of clinical disorders.

Today, more and more new laboratory tests are employed to arrive at the final diagnosis of clinical disorders. An understanding of these various methods provides the student, the physicians and medical practitioners, a useful guide for the correct applications and interpretation of results thereby leading to correct diagnosis, appropriate use of drug, patients assurance, treatment and relief.

In the second part of this book, the various tests for the detection of viruses and their products in clinical samples are discussed.

Attempts will be made to make it as practical as possible for the maximum benefit of the reader.

Serological Assays for the detection of viral antigen-antibody reactions

Serology is the measurement and characterisation of antibodies, antigens and other immunological substance in body fluids, usually after viral infection.

Diagnosis of viral infection by measuring the immune response to the virus infection became a landmark in diagnostic virology. Serology remains an important tool in the diagnosis of acute viral infection especially when virus isolation is difficult, as well as for the determination of specific antiviral immunity. Following exposure to viruses, the host immune system is capable of mounting a response in form of antibody production. Antiviral antibodies become detectable in the serum weeks after such exposure. The kinetic of such antibody response forms the basis of serological response as a diagnostic tool. Immunoglobulin M (IgM) is usually the first to appear in the serum following infection and the first to disappear. The level of IgM may peak within the first one month, but steadily declines within 2 months. However, low level may remain for about a year or more. IgG appears almost at the same period, peaks gradually and persists for a very long time as long as the lifetime of the individual. Thus, presence of IgM in the serum is a sign of current infection while IgG signifies past exposure or immunity due to vaccination.

Serological diagnosis of acute infection is precipitated on the immunological changes taking place in the host serum. This change is usually in the form of seroconversion, which may consist of absence of viral specific antibody at acute phase but presence of same weeks later at the convalescent phase sera and the presence of IgM at acute phase. The presence of IgM in the acute phase is very important because it allows early diagnosis and intervention.

Presence of virus specific antibodies in some acute diseases like measles and rubella are diagnostic, and typical of past infection, but in some chronic diseases like HIV, HTLV, and hepatitis, the presence of these antibodies usually point to a current active infection. This is particularly important in the screening tests for HIV and hepatitis that have become so important in the early diagnosis of these diseases and in the screening of blood for blood transfusion.

Serological tests are very important for defining population immunity and for monitoring vaccination programme. Today, there are very sensitive serological methods like the enzyme immunosorbent assays (EIA) that can measure antibody in their micro concentration. This is particularly important as antibody level declines with time after infection.

Serological tests can be divided into three categories, some of the tests however being found in two of three categories:

1. Those that measure directly the interaction of antigens with antibodies(RIA, EIA, IF etc).
2. Those that depend on the capacity of antibody upon interaction with antigen to perform some non-viral related functions(HA/HI, CFT etc).
3. Those that measure directly the capacity of antibody to block some specific viral functions e.g. Neutralization test, PRNT, NI).

Immunodifussion and electroimmunodifussion

Although there are many more sensitive tests for detecting viral antigen antibody reactions today, the immunodiffusion test will continue to find its relevance in the diagnosis of viral diseases as the method is still in widespread use and has many more application in the detection and analysis of precipitating antigen antibody reaction.

The immunodiffusion test is the simplest and most direct means of demonstrating antigen antibody reaction. It detects antigen antibody complex by precipitation reaction through the formation of a lattice between the antigen determinants and the combining site of the antibody. For a precipitation to be formed, the antigen and antibody must be in the relative concentration, while the buffer electrolytes must be in the appropriate concentration to provide the needed pH and temperature. Precipitation will only form in area of equivalence between the antigen and the antibody. The test is quantitative, but can also be used as a semi-quantitative test.(Fig. 7.1)

Oudin in 1946 first described the single diffusion in agar followed by Ouchterlony's classical description of the double diffusion in agar. The test can be done in a Petri dish (macro) or in a microscope slide (micro).

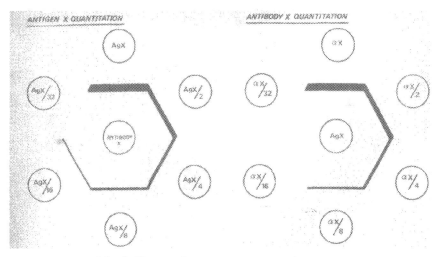

Fig. 7.1 Double diffusion for qauntitation of antigens/antibodies

Ouchterlony double diffusion in agar

Prepare a 1% agar by adding 1gm of agar into 100ml of PBS buffer pH 7.0-8.5.

Boil the suspension until the agar is molten.

Using a 5 or 10ml pipette, add about 3ml of the molten agar into the Petri dish or 0.5ml unto the microscope slide.

Allow to solidify.

Using a well puncher, punch a 3-4mm diameter well in the centre and 4-6 surrounding wells around the central well depending on the number of the samples.

Using a Pasteur pipette, fill the center well with the antigen.

Using another Pasteur pipette, fill the upper and lower wells with a known positive antiserum to the antigen.

Fill the remaining side wells with the test sera.

Incubate the agar wells in moist chamber at 37°C overnight or at room temperature for about 24-48 hours.
Check for precipitin lines.

Depending on the types of precipitin lines formed, the lines can either be line of identify, non-identify or partial identify.
The position of precipitin lines between the central and surrounding antibody wells is proportional to the relative concentration of the reagents. If the concentration of antibody is in relative excess over the antigen, the precipitin line will form closer to the antigen well and vice-versa.

Some interpretation
If two different antigens are present and can be recognised by a given antibody, two independent lines of precipitation will form on the agar. (Fig 7.2).

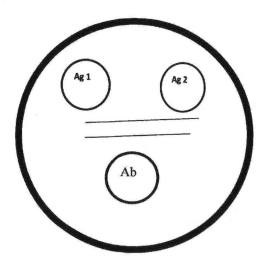

Fig. 7.2 Two separate antigens recognised by a single antibody

It is possible to distinguish separate antigen-antibody reaction if produced by different populations of antibody present in the serum.

The Outchterlony method can therefore be used to determine the relationship between antigens and a particular test antibody.

For example, in reaction I shown below(Fig 7.3), precipitin lines are formed between the antibody and the two antigens indicating that the antibody is precipitating identical epitopes in each preparation i.e epitope 1. This does not mean that the antigens are necessarily identical but they are all identical as far as the antibody can differentiate the difference.

In reaction II, (Fig 7.4) the antibody preparation distinguishes the 3 different antigens. Lines of non-identities were formed.

In reaction III, (Fig 7.5) the antigens share epitope 1, but one antigen also has epitope 2. The antibody can distinguish the two different antigens by virtue of being able to react against both epitopes. A line of identity forms with anti-epitope 1 with the addition of a spur where the anti-epitope 2 has reacted with the second epitope.

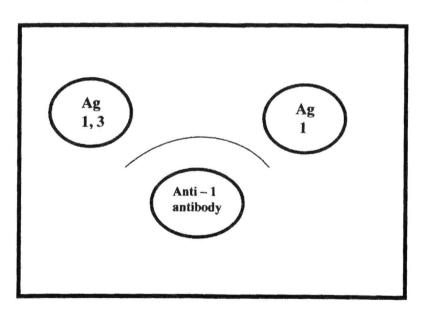

Fig. 7.3. Precipitin lines of identity

II

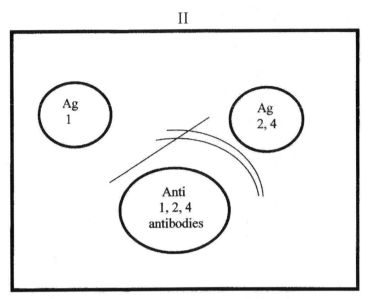

Fig 7.4 showing lines of non-identity as a result of the antibody
preparation distinguishing the 3 different antigens

III

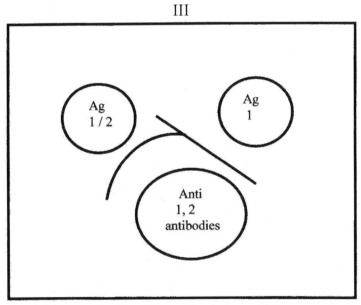

Fig 7.5 showing line of identity with epitope 1 and partial identity
with epitope 2. Note the formation of a spur towards the
cross-reacting antigen.

Single Radial immunodiffusion

The single radial immunodiffusion is a semiquantitative test based on the principle that a quantitative relationship exists between the amount of antigen put in a well cut in an agar-antibody plate and the resulting ring of precipitation. This method was first described by Mancini in 1965.

Procedure

Fill a Petri dish with 3 ml of semisolid agar to which antiserum A has been mixed.

Allow to solidify (15-20 minutes) and with a gel puncher, punch a well in the centre.

Fill the centre well with a measured amount of an antigen homolgous to the antibody.

Incubate in a moist chamber at room temperature or at 37⁰C for 24-48 hours during which time the antigen is allowed to diffuse radially.

5. Where the antigen forms an equivalent concentration with the antibody in the agar, a precipitin line will be formed.

To quantitate an amount of antigen.

Make a serial dilution of the antigen starting with the undiluted to a desired dilution.

7. Punch corresponding wells in the agar-antiserum well.

8. Fill the wells with the serially diluted antigens. For the final determination of the concentration of the unknown antigens, one of the wells must be filled with a standardised antigen.

Incubate in a moist chamber as before.

At the completion of diffusion, rings with diameters corresponding to the concentration of the antigen will form around the wells.

The ring diameters should be measured across the rings with a metre rule from the edges of each ring.

Calculate the amount of unknown antigen by comparison with standard.

A standard curve showing the relationship between ring diameter and antigen concentration is used to determine the concentration of the antigen.

The size of the ring is proportional to the initial concentration of antigen. The radial immunodiffusion test permits semi-quantitation of antigen or antibody. The initial concentration of the antigen can be calculated using the formula.

$$\text{Log } C = \frac{D - Do}{K}$$

where   C = antigen concentration
             Do = intercept with ordinate
             D = ring diameter
             K = slope of line.

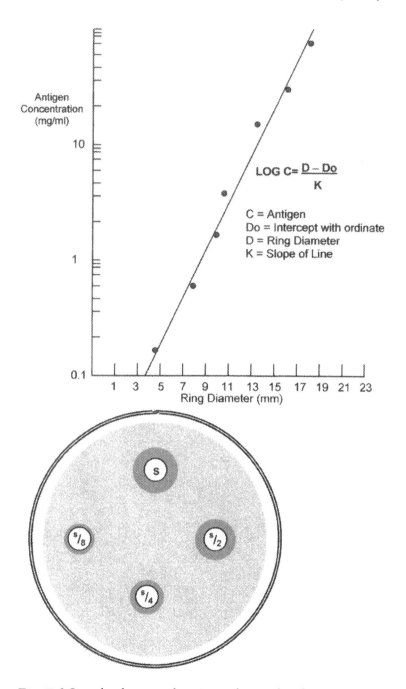

Fig. 7.6 Standard curve showing relationship between ring
diameter and antigen concentration.

Immuno Electrophoresis

The immunoelectrophoresis method combined electrophoresis and precipitation in agar to get a simple but powerful method for identifying antigens in complexes using the property of protein's (antigen's) ability to separate into positive and negative polarity in an electrical field with agar or cellulose acetate acting as a stabilising medium. In the ordinary immunodiffusion, antigen and antibody are allowed to come into contact and precipitate in agar purely by diffusion. The chance of antigen and antibody meeting and the speed of development of precipitation line can be greatly enhanced by electrically driving the two reagents towards each other.

Immunoelectrophoresis can be performed as follows:

Unto a glass slide pour about 0.3 ml of agar or agarose in a buffer solution (pH 8.2).

Allow to solidify.

Punch an antigen well in the centre and an antiserum trough at the top.

Fill the well with antigen and allow to separate in an electrical field for 30-60 minutes. The antigen will migrate according to its electrophoretic mobility.

Fill the antiserum trough with the antibody and allow to diffuse for 18-24 hours.

Precipitin lines will form according to the different epitopes in the antigen recognised by the antiserum.

Precipitin lines showing lines of identify, partial identify or non-identify will be formed (Fig 7.7).

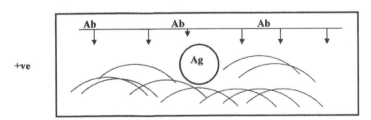

Fig 7.7 – Immunoelectrophoresis in a microscope slide showing different antigen/antibody reactions.

Numerous variations of the electroimmunodiffusion have been described. Only one will be described here i.e. The One dimensional double electroimmunodiffusion variation which is demonstrated by the counter immnoelectrophoresis (CIEOP), also known as counter current electrophoresis.

Counter Immunoelectrophoresis (CIEOP).

This is also known as Countercurrent electrophoresis.

This is an electrodiffussion technique in which antigen and the antibody driven by electric current from opposite direction meet each other. The antigen well must be on the left and cathodal (-ve) end while the antibody is placed on the right and anodal (+ve) end of the agarose gel slide. The pH of the agarose buffer must be such as to make the antibody positively charged while the antigen is negatively charged. The antibody is driven towards the antigen by an electrophorectic force while the antibody is driven towards the antigen by an electroendoosmosis force.

Procedure

1. Make a 1% agarose in borate saline buffer solution pH 8.0-8.2.
2. Pipette 0.3ml of the molten agarose on a clean microscope slide and allow to solidify.
3. Punch a well on both ends of the slide to be equidistant from the centre of the well.
4. Mark the slide to indicate anode (+ve) and cathode (-ve) ends of the slide.
5. Fill the anodal well with the antigen and the cathodal well with the antiserum.
6. Fill the electrophoretic jar with electrophoretic buffer consisting of borate buffer solution pH 9.2, and carefully place the slide such that the electrophoretic buffer covers the slide slightly.
7. Align the polarity of the jar to correspond with the polarity of the slide.

8. Connect the jar to a power pack and run at 60-65 volts for 2 hours.(Fig. 7.8)

Precipitin line will form within 30 minutes. The CIEOP is about 10 times more sensitive than the standard double diffusion techniques.

Some of the antigens that can be detected by the CIEOP include HBsAg, cyptococcal specific antigens, meniccococal specific antigens, haemophillus specific antigens carcinoembryonic antigen, cord IgM, Alpha$_1$fetoprotein and dermatophilosis virus of cattle.

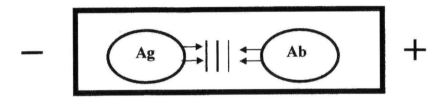

Fig 7.8 Counterimmunoelectrophoresis

Haemagglutination and Haemagglutination Inhibition Test

Certain group of viruses possesses in their outer envelopes glycoproteins called haemagglutinins which are capable of agglutinating erythrocytes. These haemagglutinins also produce haemagglutinating antibodies when in contact with immunocompetent hosts. The presence of these haemagglutins and heamaglutinating antibodies can therefore be used to identify these groups of viruses in clinical samples as well as determine haemaglutinating antibodies titre of sera from hosts. Most of the haemagglutinating viruses are in the Orthomyxoviridae and Paramyxoviridae families- influenza and measles viruses- although other viruses like adenovirus, rubella virus, arboviruses, mumps virus, reoviruses and some enteroviruses also possess haemagglutins which will haemagglutinate red blood cells (RBC).

Different haemagglutinating viruses will cause haemagglutination of different animal RBCs. For example, measles virus will only haemagglutinate monkey RBC and some human group O RBC while influenza virus will haemagglutinate chicken RBC. The principle of the Haemagglutination-inhibition test (HI) is based on the ability of the haemagglutinating antibody in serum binding with the antigen (in this case the virus) and therefore not making it available to agglutinate RBC thus indicating previous exposure of the host to the virus.

Although the HI test is not as sensitive as the EIA, it is still finding wide application in those diagnostic laboratories where the EIA are not available, and in the identification of new isolates of some viruses.

Before running the HI test, the HA test must first of all be run to determine the HA titre of the virus or viral antigen, from which the challenge antigen will be calculated.

HI test can often be complicated by the presence of non-specific inhibitors and agglutinins in the serum. This must be removed to avoid false positive or false negative results. Removal of these inhibitors or haemagglutinins is by treating the test sera with Kaolin and RBC absorption(measles virus), receptor-destroying enzyme (RDE) treatment (influenza virus) and heat inactivation or potassium periodate treatment(adenovirus). For virus identification, a known virus-specific antiserum must be used, and for antibody titre determination, a known virus antigen must be used.

Procedure for HI test
Materials needed

Blood from avian, monkey, guinea pig (depending on the type of virus)

Alsevers solution

PBS 0.01M pH7.2

U or V bottom 96-well microtitre plates

Dilution loops or micropipette tips

Single and multichannel micopipettes, 100 ml, 200 ml or 1000 ml.

Reading mirror

Water bath or incubator

RBC Preparation (Measles virus)

Procedure

1. Obtain about 5 ml of blood in Alsevers solution from the African green monkey through the femoral vein. The animal must be well restrained.
2. Mix thoroughly with 5 ml of PBS and spin at 3000 rpm for 10 minutes. Pour away the supernantant.
3. Repeat the washing two more times with 10 ml of PBS and pour off the supernantant.
4. Determine the packed cell volume and make a 10% suspension from the packed cell (V/V) in PBS. This can keep for a week at 2-8^{0}C.
5. Prepare the desired concentration (vol/vol) from the 10% stock on the day of the test.

Haemagglutination Test

Procedure

1. Make a 1:2 dilution of the antigen in a tube and dispense 100µl in the first well of the first two rows of the 96 well plates.
2. Add 50µl of PBS or normal saline to all the wells of the first two rows of the U or V bottom 96-well plate starting from the second well.
3. Using a 100µl micropipette with tip, remove 50µl of the antigen from the first well into the second well. Pipette gently up and down to dilute.
4. Changing the tip after every other dilution, repeat the two-fold dilution process until the 10th well and discard the last 50µl. This will give a dilution of 1:2 to 1:1024. Leave the remaining two wells for RBC control.
5. Add 50µl of the 0.8% RBC into all the wells including the RBC control wells.
6. Incubate at 4°C overnight or at 37^{0}C for 1 hour. Read the test and record. The optimum time to read the test

is often guided by the time there is formation of distinct button in the RBC control wells.

The titre of the antigen is the reciprocal of the dilution when there is complete agglutination of the RBC. That dilution contains 1HA unit in the well.

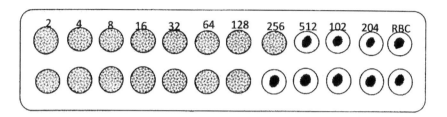

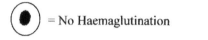 = No Haemaglutination   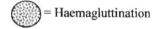 = Haemagluttination

Fig.7.9 Haemagglutination Test

In the example in Fig 7.9, the titre of the antigen is 128 HA Units/50µl. This means at a dilution of 1: 128, there is 1 Haemagglutination Unit/50µl of the antigen.

Haemagglutination Inhibition Test for Virus Identification

For virus identification, a type specific antiserum for the suspected virus must be available. The standard virus dilution for running the HI test is 4HA unit of the antigen.

Procedure

1. *Cal*culate the 4 HA unit from the titre of the antigen obtained from the HA test by dividing the titre by 4. From the example above, the titre of the antigen is 128; the dilution that will contain 4 HA unit is 1:32. This is made by mixing 1ml of the undiluted antigen and 31ml or 0.1ml in 3.1ml of PBS.

2. *Mak*e 2-fold serial dilution of the type-specific antiserum in U or V bottom 96-well plate starting from 1:2 in 50µl volume.
3. *Add* 50µl of the antigen containing the 4HA unit. Gently tap the edges of the plate for a few seconds to allow the antigen and the antiserum to mix.
4. Incubate at 37°C for 1 hour.
5. Add 50µl of the 0.8% monkey RBC and incubate overnight at 4°C or 1 hour at 37°C.
6. Do a back titration to check and confirm that the correct unit of antigen was used:
   (a). In the same 96-well plate, add 50µl of PBS into the wells starting from the 2nd to the 6th well.
7. (b). Add 100ul of the dilution containing the 4 HA unit into the first well of the same row.
   (c). Take 50µl of the 4 HA unit from the first well into the second well and mix thoroughly. Repeat the dilution until the 6th well and discard the last 50µl.
8. Add 50µl of the 0.8% RBC to all the wells.
9. Incubate the plate at 4°C overnight. Plate may also be incubated at 37°C for 1 hour. For haemagglutinating viruses containing neuraminidase, it is advisable that the result be read in time before elution.

If the right HA unit was used, haemagglutination will be observed in the first 3 wells of the back titration wells while in the test wells inhibition of heamagglutination will be observed in those wells where the type specific serum has reacted with the antigen and thus not making it available to heamagglutinate the antigen. The titre of the serum is the highest dilution showing complete inhibition of heamagglutination of the monkey RBC. Titres of type-specific antiserum equal to or higher than 1:160 is regarded as positive and identifies the virus.

Haemagglutination Test for Antibody Determination

The HI test can be used to determine antibody levels in sera. In this case a known type-specific antigen must be available. Sera must be heat-inactivated at 56°C for 30 minutes and treated to remove non-specific inhibitors and agglutinins. Sera heated longer may lead to false positive result. The treatment of sera for different viruses are described in the next page.

Procedure

1. Make a 2-fold serial dilution of the sera in 96 well plates in 50ul volume in PBS. (These sera should include acute phase, covalescent phase, known negative and known positive sera).

2. Add 50µl of the 4 HA units into all the wells containing serum dilution. Do the back titration for the virus control and leave some well without antigen for RBC control. Incubate plate at 37°C for 1 hour.

3. Add 50ul of the 0.8% into all the wells. Incubate overnight at 4°C or at 37°C for 1 hour.

4. Read the result.

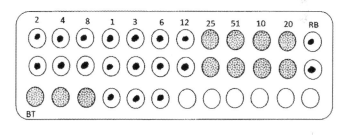

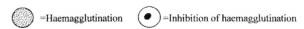

Fig 7.10 Haemagglutination inhibition test for the identification of virus or determination of antiserum titre.

In the example above, the titre of the serum is 128. The test is valid because the virus control well represented in the third row shows that the correct 4 HA unit was used and the RBC control in wells 12 of the first two rows show no sign of heamagglutination.

The acute phase and negative sera should show low or no antiserum titre while the positive control and convalescent sera should give a high level titre. For diagnostic purposes, a 4-fold or greater rise between the acute and covalescent phase sera is suggestive of recent infection by the test virus.

The HI test can be used to determine the herd immunity of a population and seroconversion rate following vaccination programme.

The advantages of HAI tests are that they are relatively easy and inexpensive to perform. The disadvantages are that HAI tests are not as sensitive as EIAs, the actual reading of results is subjective and the reagents should be fresh or else abnormal agglutination patterns may arise which makes the reading and interpretation of the test very difficult. As a result the HAI test for some viruses had been replaced by more sensitive and reliable EIA tests for IgG in many virus diagnostic laboratories.

Preparation of High Potent Measles Haemagglutinating Antigen

Experience has shown in our laboratory that measles virus isolated in tissue culture is not potent enough to haemagglutinate, even after sonication or other physical treatment.

Therefore measles antigen was prepared by ether extraction.

Procedure:
1. Grow Vero cell in T 150 tissue culture flask in 10% Minimum Essential Medium (MEM).
2. After attaining confluency, inoculate 0.4 ml of measles virus (The Edmonson vaccine strain) and incubate at 37°C. Two days post inoculation, change the culture medium to maintainance medium supplemented with 2% fetal calf serum. This stage is very important to achieve highly potent antigen.
3. Examine cells daily for measles specific CPE. Harvest the cells when the CPE is about 80-90%.

4. Freeze thaw the infected cells in 3 cycles at -70°C, and further break the cells into smaller units by pipetting up and down.

5. Spin at low speed centrifugation, 3000 rpm for 10 minutes to clear the debris.

6. Pour the supernatant into a clean sterile 50ml centrifutge tube.

7. Concentrate the virus fluid with 60% PEG at a final concentration of 10% and keep at 40°C overnight. The following day, spin at 8000 rpm for 1 hour.

8. Add Tween 80 at a final concentration of 0.125-0.3 % and shake vigourously for a few minutes.

9. Add half volume of ether and shake for about 15 minutes on ice.

10. Centrifuge at 3000 rpm for 20 minutes.

11. Remove residual ether by bubbling through nitrogen. In the absence of nitrogen, pour the antigen in a sterile Petri dish. Place under a lamina flow hood with the blower overnight.

12. Test the antigen for heamagglunination activity.

Treatment of Sera for HI Test

Human sera contain some non-specific inhibitors and agglutinins which may complicate the results of haemagglutation. These must be removed to achieve a reliable result.

Receptor-Destroying Enzyme (RDE)

Sera for testing of anti-influenza antibodies must be treated with RDE.

Procedure

1. Add 0.4 ml of RDE to 0.1 ml of serum and incubate at 37°C overnight.

2. Add 0.3 ml of 2.5% sodium citrate and heat at 56°C for 30 minutes.

3. Add 0.2 ml of PBS. This will give a final dilution of the serum of 1:10.

Kaolin Treatment

Kaolin is used for the treatment of sera for measles and yellow fever virus heamaglutination or compliment fixation tests.

Procedure
1. Prepare a 25% suspension of Kaolin (acid-wash) in PBS.
2. Dilute the serum 1:5 in PBS and mix with equal volume of the Kaolin suspension.
3. Shake vigorously and allow to stand at room temperature for 20 minutes. Shake intermittently.
4. Centrifuge at 2000 rpm for 30 minutes.

The supernatant is a 1:10 dilution of the original serum.

Trypsin and Periodate Treatment

1. Mix 0.1 ml of 0.8% Trypsin solution in PBS with 0.2ml of undiluted serum and alow to stand at 56°C for 30 minutes.
2. Add 0.6ml of 0.01M aqueous potassium periodate solution (225gm/100ml distilled water). Allow to stand at room temperature for 15 minutes.
3. Add 0.6ml of 1% aqueous glycerol solution and allow to stand for additional 15 minutes at room temperature.
4. Add 0.5ml PBS to arrive at a final dilution of 1:10.

Removal of non-specific Agglutinin

Apart from the non-specific inhibitors, certain sera contain natural agglutinins against erythrocytes. After inactivation and removal of non-specific inhibitors, such sera must be treated by absorption with RBC to remove these agglutinins.

Procedure
1. Add 0.1 ml of 50% washed RBC to 1ml of the already treated sera. Allow to stand inside the refrigerator for 60 minutes.

2. Centrifuge at 4°C at 1,500 rpm for 10 minutes.

The supernantant contains the sera at a concentration of 1:10.

Complement Fixation Test

The Complement Fixation Test (CFT) is a very useful serological test for the detection of virus isolates in clinical samples and for the determination of antibody levels in large number of serum. It is a simple but yet commonly used test. However the test has the limitation of being group-specific and will not be able to detect type-specific antigens from the viral group. Successful performance of the CFT depends to a large extents on the standardisation of all the reagents to be used and the level of experience of the person performing the test.

Like any other antigen/antibody reaction, the CFT depends on the interaction of antigen, antibody and complement. The principle of the test is predicated on the ability of antigen and antibody combining together to form a complex and bind/fix complement. Neither antigen nor antibody on its own will bind/fix complement. A bound/fixed complement will not be available to lyse haemolysin sensitised sheep red blood cell which is the indicator system of the test. This will indicate a positive test result. When the antigen and the antibody do not form complex, the complement is not bound/fixed and therefore available to lyse the sensitised sheep red blood cell. This will indicate a negative result.

(1) **Ag + Ab – Ag/Ab Complex + C' – AgAbC'**

AgAbC' + RBC = No Lysis (Positive Test)

(2) **Ag + Ab ≠ Ag +Ab + C' – Ag, Ab, C'**

Ag, Ab, C' + RBC – Lysis (Negative Test)

The CFT comprises two stages i.e. the antigen/antibody reaction stage and the indicator stage made up of sheep red blood cell and heamolysin.

List of Materials
Sheep red blood cell
Rabbit antibody to sheep red blood cells (hemolysin)
Guinea pig serum (source of complement)
U- or V-bottom 96-well microtitre plates
Veronal Buffer Stock Solution
Solution A

NaCl	83.80g
$NaHCO_3$	2.52g
Sodium barbital (sodium 5,5-diethyl barbiturate	3.00
Deionised Distilled H_2O	1000 ml

Solution B

Barbital (5,5-diethyl barbituric acid)	4.60g
$MgCl_2$	1.00g
$CaCl_2.2H_2O$	0.20g
Hot Distilled deionised H_2O	500ml

Allow both solutions to cool and thereafter add solution A to solution B and make up to a total volume of 2000ml with distilled water. This will give a 5X stock solution. Sterilize by filtration. A 1:5 dilution of the buffer should be used as the working dilution.

Standardization of reagents
Prior to performing the test, all the reagents must be standardised.

Heamolysin dilution and red blood cell sensitisation
The sheep red blood cells must be sensitised by incubating it with haemolysin. Haemolysin is obtained by inoculating rabbit with sheep

red blood cell. A stock solution of haemolysin can be prepared at a 1:100 concentration and stored at -20°C.

Procedure:

Make from the 1:100 stock of haemolysin a 1:1000 to 1:40,000 dilution in Veronal buffer.

Add equal volume of a 2% washed sheep red blood cell to each dilution and incubate at 37°C for 30 minutes. This will sensitize the sheep red blood cell.

Dilution of Heamolysin	Heamolysin solution 1:1000 (ml)	Veronal Buffer (ml)	Discard excess (ml)	Heamolysin Final volume (ml)	2% sheep red blood cell (ml)
1:1000	2.0	-	-	2.0	2.0
1:2000	1.0	1.0		2.0	2.0
1:4000	0.5	1.5		2.0	2.0
1:6000	0.4	2.0	0.4	2.0	2.0
1:8000	0.3	2.1	0.4	2.0	2.0
1:10000	0.2	1.8		2.0	2.0
1:15000	0.2	2.8	1.0	2.0	2.0
1:20000	0.2	3.8	2.0	2.0	2.0
1:30000	0.2	5.8	4.0	2.0	2.0
1:40000	0.2	7.8	6.0	2.0	2.0

Table 7.1: Preparation of Heamolysin Dilution and sensitisation of sheep RBC

Standardisation of Complement Units

The source of complement is the guinea pig sera. It must however be tested for the absence of antibody to the antigen to be tested. A stock solution of complement prepared at a concentration of 1:10 in veronal buffer is prepared and kept on ice during the test period.

Procedure:

Make a dilution starting from 1:50 to 1:240 as shown in the Table 7.2 from the 1:10 stock solution.

Add 0.2 ml of the sensitised sheep RBC to 0.2 ml of the various complement dilutions with the serial dilution of heamolysin starting from 1:1000 as shown in the Table 7.2

Add 0.2 ml of cold veronal buffer to each mixture and incubate for 1 hour at 37oC. It can also be incubated overnight at 4°C.

Read and record the highest dilution of complement that gives 100% hemolysis. The highest dilution of complement at a heamolysin dilution giving 100% represents 1 unit of the complement. Generally for identifying viruses, 2 full units of complement should be used.

Heamolysin dilutions with sensitised RBC	Complement Dilutions													Veronal Buffer only
	50	60	70	80	90	100	120	140	160	180	200	220	240	
1:1000	0	0	0	0	0	0	0	0	0	0	2	2	4	4
1:2000	0	0	0	0	0	0	0	0	0	0	2	2	4	4
1:4000	0	0	0	0	0	0	0	0	0	0	2	2	4	4
1:6000	0	0	0	0	0	0	2	2	4	4	4	4	4	4
1:8000	0	0	0	0	0	0	2	4	4	4	4	4	4	4
1:10000	0	0	0	1	2	2	4	4	4	4	4	4	4	4
1:15000	0	1	2	2	2	4	4	4	4	4	4	4	4	4
1:20000	4	4	4	4	4	4	4	4	4	4	4	4	4	4
1:30000	4	4	4	4	4	4	4	4	4	4	4	4	4	4
1:40000	4	4	4	4	4	4	4	4	4	4	4	4	4	4

0 =Complete or 100% heamolysis
1 =75% heamolysis
2 = 50% heamolysis
3 = 25% heamolysis
4 = No heamolysis

Table 7.2 showing example of determination of complement units

In this test, a heamolysin dilution of 1:4000 and a complement dilution of 1:180 completely heamolysed the sensitised sheep RBC. Therefore at a 1:4000 heamolysin dilution, 1:180 complement contains 1 unit of complement.
1:90 contains 2 Units
1:45 contains 4 Units.
To run the test with 2 Units, one part of complement is added to 89 parts of veronal buffer.

Complement fixation test for the identification of virus isolate
After all the reagents have been standardised, the test proper can now be performed.

The CFT test is usually performed in a 96- well microtitre plate. The plate should be marked as shown in Fig 7.11.

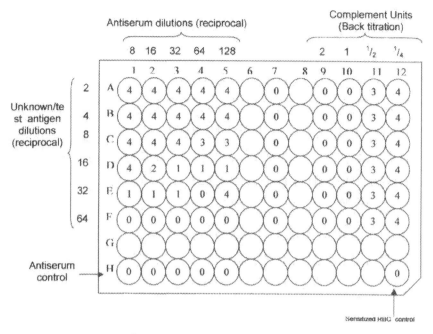

Fig 7.11 Complement Fixation Test for the identification
of virus isolate

Procedure
1. Dispense 25μl of veronal buffer to wells 2-5 of rows A-F and H.
2. Add 25ul of 1:10 antiserum dilution to each well 1 and 2 of rows A-F and H.
3. Make serial 2-fold dilutions of the antiserum from wells 2-5 of row A. Repeat this in row B-F and H for antiserum controls.
4. Make a two fold dilution of the unknown antigen starting from 1:2 to 1:64.
5. Transfer 25μl of each antigen dilution to wells 1-5 containing anitesum dilution and well 7 for antigen controls, starting from the highest antigen dilution to the lowest, ie row F back to A.

6. Add 25ul veronal buffer to row H wells(antiserum control) and column 7 wells (antign controls).

7. Dilute complement in cold veronal buffer to contain 2 units in 25ul.

8. Add 25ul of the complement dilution to all the wells.

9. Gently mix by tapping the plate, avoiding any spill from the well.

10. Do a back titration of the complement by adding veronal buffer to wells 10-12 of rows A-F.

11. Add 25ul containing 2 units of the complement to well in columns 9 and 10 in rows A-F.

12. Make serial 2-fold dilution of complement in columns 10-12 of row A, to contain 1, ½ and ¼ unit. Repeat same in rows B-F.

13. Add 25ul of each unknown antigen dilution starting from the highest to the lowest dilution to wells 9-12 from rows F back to A.

14. Do the RBC control by adding 75ul veronal buffer to well 12 of row H.

15. Seal the plate and incubate overnight at 4-6oC.

Procedures 1-15 complete the antigen/antibody stage. The next stage is the indicator stage which is by the addition of sensitised sheep RBC.

16. Remove plate from the refrigerator and bring up to room temperature. This will take about 15-30 minutes.

17. Meanwhile, prepare sensitised sheep RBC by adding equal amount of 1.4% sheep RBC to heamolysin which had been diluted to contain 2 units in 25ul. Incubate at 37^0C for 30 minutes.

18. Add 50ul of the sensitised sheep RBC to each well.

19. Shake plate gently to mix.

20. Incubate at 37oC for 15-30 minutes or until the antigen control shows complete heamolysis. Allow the unlysed RBC to settle.

Read the results by observing the degree of heamolysis in the various wells scoring the heamolysis as follows:

    0 = Complete heamolysis (No fixation= Negative)
    1 = 75% heamolysis
    2 = 50% heamolysis
    3 = 25% heamolysis
    4 = No heamolysis(Complete fixation=Positive)

The highest dilution of antigen showing 4+ fixation with the highest dilution of antiserum indicates the identity of the virus in relation to the known antiserum.

Test is not valid if there is fixation in any of the antigen or antiserum wells.

Interpretation of test

The CFT is based on the interaction between the antigen, antibody and complement. Therefore, when the test is used for virus identification, complete fixation, i.e no heamolysis, at moderate to high dilution of the unknown antigen shows close identity of the virus while complete fixation at low dilution of the unknown antigen could be a non-specific reaction. If the test is used for antibody level determination, complete fixation at the highest serum dilution indicates the end point of the serum and as such the titre of the serum.

The Complement Fixation Test has some advantages and disadvantages. The advantages include ability to screen against a large number of viral infections at the same time. It is also cheap to run because there is no need for expensive equipment. These advantages are almost dwarfed by the disadvantages, chief among which are its low sensitivity which may not make the test a good test for immunity screening. It is time consuming and labour intensive. It is often non-specific, often giving reactions between cross reacting viruses.

Immunohistochemical Methods

To the immunohistochemical assay belong two serological methods – the immunofluorescent (IF) staining technique and the immunoperoxidase (IP) staining. Both methods are used for the direct detection of antigens in clinical specimens and antibodies in virus-cell systems. The principles of both tests are almost the same. The IP, however, is more cumbersome to run but has some advantages over the IF method. The stained specimen can be viewed in IP directly by a light miscrope or naked eyes instead of a fluorescent microscope which may not be easily available in most virology laboratories. Reagents are most stable. The development of high-quality monoclonal antibodies to a variety of viruses today has made the use of IF and IP more routine in many laboratories and have contributed to the rapid detection of these viruses in clinical specimens. Specific identification can be made within hours of staining or CPE detection.

Immunofluorescent Technique (IFT)

The principle of the IFT is based on the ability of the antigen or antibody binding with a fluorescent marker usually fluorescein isothiocyanete, (FITC) and yet retaining its abilities to bind with the antibody or antigen (reactivity). There are two methods – the direct method for detecting viral antigens and the indirect method for detecting antibodies. The direct method is simpler and quicker, while the indirect method is more sensitive and widely applicable and requires only one conjugate for the detection of a variety of antigen-antibody reactions as long as all the virus-specific antibodies are produced in a single animal species. The IF is readily used for the detection of viral antigens in autopsy tissues, histopathological tissues and viral infected tissue culture cells. There are commercially available welled-slides for IF tests today for rapid test.

List of materials and reagents
Miscrope slides
Acetone
Known positive antigen/antiserum
Flourescent microscope
Flouroscein isothiocyanate(FITC)
PBS buffer, glycerine buffer
Virus infected cells showing CPE
Capillary pipettes

Slide Preparation

Procedure

1. Clean the slide thoroughly and allow to dry.
2. Depending on the clinical specimen, this can be tissue or cell, mince or disrupt cells/tissues and resuspend in PBS such that they contain enough cell suspensions.
3. Place a drop of the cells containing suspected antigen into each of the well of 8 or 12 welled slide. Prepare enough well sufficient for the test.
4. Allow to air dry at room temperature.
5. Fix the cells in cold acetone for 10 minutes and again air dry. Store away slides at -20°C until ready for use. Avoid moisturising the stored slides.
6. Prepare some positive and negative slides as controls. A positive slide can be made from a tissue culture cell line infected with a known virus and which is showing CPE while a negative slide is made from the same cell line but not infected with virus.

Direct IFT for Ag-Detection

Procedure

1. Prior to running the test, remove slides from -20°C and allow to equilibrate at room temperature.
2. Overlay cell spots on slide with fluorescein-labelled specific antibody to the suspected virus. Incubate slides at 37°C for 30 minutes, or at room temperature in a moist chamber.
3. Wash cells spots with PBS three times to remove excess labelled antibody. Air dry slide at room temperature.
4. Mount the slides with glycerine buffer: 1 ml PBS + 9 ml glycerine.
5. Cover with a microscope slide.
6. Examine the slides under the IF microscope with a dark-field condenser and a UV light source.

If the antigen in the slide is specific for the labelled antibody, an apple green fluorescence will be seen under the microscope while the surrounding cells will stain deep red or brown.

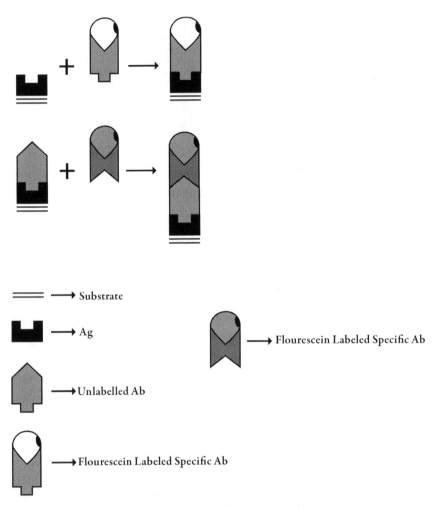

Fig. 7.12 Direct Method for antigen detection
by immuofluorescent technique

Indirect IF for Antibody Detection

This is usually referred to as the "sandwiched" method. The antiviral antibody to be detected is unlabelled and is detected by a second antibody that binds to immunoglobulins from the specimen of origin of the first antibody (usually anti-mouse) because most of monoclonal antibodies are prepared from mice. This second antibody which is referred to as the detector is conjugated with the fluorescein marker. In this case the unlabelled antibody plays the role of antibody in the primary reaction and antigen in the secondary reaction.

Procedure

1. Overlay cell spots on slides (to which the antigen had been previously fix-dried)with the unlabelled antiserum (test serum) or monoclonal antibody.
2. Allow to stand for 30 minutes at room temperature in a petri dish in a humid chamber.
3. Wash off excess antibody three times with PBS and allow to air dry at room temperature.
4. Add the detector immunoglobulin i.e the fluorescein-labelled goat anti-mouse immunoglobulin to the cell spots on slides and allow for 30 minutes to react with the unlabelled monoclonal antibody or test antibody that was added in step 1. Wash off excess labelled antiglobulin, with PBS three times and again air dry.
5. Mount slight in glycerine buffer and examine as above.

If the antibody in the unlabelled serum (test or monoclonal) is specific for the viral antigen, an apple green florescence will be observed under the microscope. In contrast, if there is no viral antigen in the original sample against the specific-unlabelled monoclonal antibody, no fluorescence will be seen.

For correct interpretation of the test, there is need for the relevant controls.

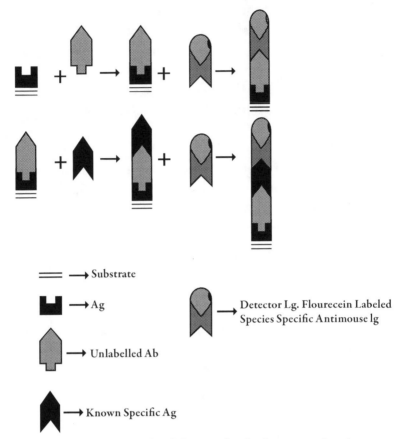

= → Substrate

▣ → Ag

◮ → Unlabelled Ab

◮ → Detector Lg. Flourecein Labeled Species Specific Antimouse lg

▲ → Known Specific Ag

Fig. 7.13 Indirect Method for antibody detection by the immunofluorescent technique

Fig.7.14: An example of a positive immunofluorescense antigen

Immunoperoxidase Staining Technique

The immunoperoxidase technique in principle is very similar to the IF. However, instead of fluorescein as marker, an enzyme is used as a conjugate. The enzyme commonly used is the horse radish peroxidase (HRP). In the direct method, a virus-specific antibody is labelled with the enzyme conjugate while in the indirect method the anti-animal species antibody is labelled. The presence of antibody/ antigen conjugate complex is detected by a substrate which can either be diaminobenzidine or sminoethylcarbazole. This is oxidised by hydrogen peroxide to yield a reddish-brown colour. The addition of the substrate is one major difference between the two tests. In the immunoperoxidase test, the substrate is a reducing agent, while the substrate in the IFA test is the base or tissue culture cells containing the antigen.

Materials and equipment
Slides and cover slides
PBS Buffer
Acetone
4% paraformaldehyde
H_2O_2 Methanol solution
Horseradish peroxidase
Xylene
50%, 70%, 90%, 100% Alcohol
0.25% Trypsin containing 0.02% $CaCl_2$
Normal mouse serum in PBS-BSA
0.5Tween 20 in 1%PBS-BSA
Goat anti-mouse immunoglobulin conjugated with peroxidase
0.05 3,3' dianno benzidine tetrachloride(DAB)
Light microscope

Procedure for Direct and Indirect Peroxidase Staining

1. Make a smear of infected cells or tissues on a cover slip and allow to air dry.

2. Wash the infected cells on the cover slip two or three times with PBS being careful not to remove the smears.

3. Fix cells or tissues with cold acetone for 10 minutes at room temperature or with 4% buffered paraformaldehyde for 20 minutes at room temperature.

4. Treat fixed infected cells/tissues with H_2O_2 methanol solution for 5 minutes. This is to remove endogenous peroxidase which may produce a false background staining.

5. For tissues embedded in paraffin staining, use xylene for 5 minutes and hydrate in 100% alcohol followed by 95%, 70% and 50% alcohol, and water twice each. Finally wash with PBS.

6. Treat with 0.25% trypsin in PBS containing 0.02% $CaCl_2$ for 30 minutes.

7. If infected cells are grown in coverslides or smeared into coverslides, steps 5 and 6 are not necessary.

8. Overlay with 1:10 or 1:20 normal mouse serum diluted in PBS-BSA for 30 minutes to block any non-specific binding. Remove excess serum by washing in PBS.

9. Add virus-specific monoclonal antibody produced in mice to the treated cells and incubate for 60 minutes at 37°C.

10. Rinse the cells with 0.5 Tween 20 in 1% PBS-BSA.

11. Add 1:50 goat anti-mouse immunoglobulin conjugated with peroxidase diluted in PBS-BSA for 30 minutes and again wash three times.

12. Add freshly prepared 0.05 3, 3^1 diannunobenzidine tetrachloride (DAB) and allow to stand for 5-10 minutes, or better still, until brown colour begins to appear.

13. Remove substrate, wash with PBS and water.

14. Dehydrate in ethanol 50%, 70%, 95% and 100% and clarify in xylene (if tissue).

15. Mount cover slip with stained cells down on microscope with a mounting fluid.

16. Examine stained preparation with light microscope.

For direct staining, steps 8 and 11 must be omitted.

Reagents Preparation

1. 3, 3¹ diaminobenzidine tetrachloride (DAB).

DAB	-	3 mg
DDH2O	-	10 ml
H_2O_2 (30%)	-	0.05 ml

2. H2O2 - Methanol solution

H_2O_2 (30%)	-	3ml
Methanol	-	97 ml

3. PBS-BSA Diluent

PBS	-	100 ml
Bovine serum albumin	-	4 gm

Enzyme Immuno Assays (EIA)

The introduction of the enzyme Immuno Assays has further improved the diagnosis of viral diseases. Viral identification in cell culture, detection of viral antigens in clinical samples and identification of viral antibodies in serum can be accomplished using assays based on the principle of enzyme immunoassays. The principle of EIA is based on the binding of antibodies with their antigens and detection of the reaction using a component conjugated with an enzyme. This enzyme subsequently acts on its specific substrate to produce a colour change the intensity of which depends on the initial quantity of antigen or antibody being measured. When the antigen-antibody reaction takes place on a solid surface, the reaction is also known as enzyme linked immunosorbent assay (ELISA). Because of its wide applicability and sensitivity, the ELISA is one of these versatile serological tests in clinical virology that has undergone many modifications and variations. Several versions have been used for antigen detection, including the antibody capture, competitive ELISA.

Today, ELISA has become one of the rapid serological tests for screening blood for HIV positivity. It is also worthy of mentioning that ELISA techniques have been developed for a variety of viruses, thus making their identification and diagnosis faster.

The general principle of the ELISA test is based on the ability of antigen or antibody binding to an enzyme while retaining its reactivity. The test involves antigen and antibody binding together in a solid face e.g. polysterene microtitre plate, and the result of the binding visualised by an enzyme acted upon by a substrate to produce a colour change. If antibodies (usually patient's serum) are to be identified, a known viral antigen is bound to the solid phase, and if antigens are to be identified, a known viral antibody, usually a monoclonal antibody is bound to the solid phase. At times the antigen can be an anti- immunoglobulin specific for the antigen. This is the "capture" antibody (see below).

The use of monoclonal antibodies has led to many improvements in ELISA systems. For example, (1) higher sensitivity which is as a result of either the selection of antibodies with an extremely high affinity, or by reduction of the height and variability of the background reaction, which makes very low concentrations of analyte more readily detectable, (2) higher specificity as a result of avoiding the presence of any antibody in the assay system with specific reactivity against non-analyte epitopes and by selecting combinations of monoclonal antibodies which may further increase specificity and finally, (3) higher practicality as a result of introducing simultaneous incubation of label, solid phase and sample without risk of "prozone effect".

Reagents and equipment
Polysterene 96 well ELISA Plates
Single and multichannel pipettes
Automatic Pipettors
ELISA Reader
ELISA Washer
Blocking buffer
Washing buffer
Coating buffer
Dilution buffer

Reagents Preparation
Coating Buffer
Carbonate-Bicarbonate Buffer (pH 9.6)

Na_2CO_3	1.59 gm
$NaH CO_3$	2.93 gm
Distilled H_2O	1000 ml

Mix well and store at 4°C for about 2 weeks.

1. Washing Buffer
PBS-Tween 20 (pH 7.6)

NaCl	8.0 gm
KH_2PO_4	0.2 gm
Na_2HPO_4	1.15 gm
Deionised water	1000 ml
Tween 20	0.50 ml

Store at 4°C

2. Dilution buffer/Blocking buffer
PBS-Tween 20 (pH 7.6)

NaCl	8.0 gm
KH_2PO_4	0.2 gm
Na_2HPO	1.15 gm
Deionized water	1000 ml
Tween 20	0.50 ml
Fetal Calf Serum	50ml(5%)

This must be prepared fresh before use.

3. Substrate buffer
Diethanolamine buffer (10%)

Diethanolamine	97 ml
$MgCl_2.6H_2O$	100 mg
Distilled water	800 ml

Add HCl 1M until the pH is 9.8
Make the volume up to 1,000 ml
Store at 4°C in the dark

Antigen Detection

This can be both direct and indirect. In both cases, viral antibody is first bound to the solid phase.

Direct

Procedure

1. Coat the plate with the viral antibody. Coated plates can be stored at 4°C until ready for use.
2. Wash the coated plate three times to remove unbound antibodies.
3. Add specimen to be tested. This should include known positive and known negative controls. Incubate at 37°C for 2 hours or 4°C overnight. Wash three times to remove any unbound antigen in the specimen.
4. Add enzyme-labelled virus specific antibody. Wash three times.
5. Add the substrate solution. The type of substrate added will depend on the type of enzyme used as conjugate. If horseradish peroxidase is used, the substrate will be ABTS or orthophenyldiamine (OPD) and if alkaline phosphotase, the substrate will be p-nitrophenyl phosphate(PNP). A redox reaction with a chromogen takes place which leads to the release of nascent oxygen which eventually leads to colour change. This colour change could either be green or yellow, depending on the type of substrate. This is represented in the chemical reaction below:

Horseradish:

$HPO + H_2O_2 \rightarrow O_2$

$O_2 + OPD = $ Yellow

$O_2 + ABTS = $ Green

6. Stop the reaction by adding 3M NaOH or H_2SO_4, depending on the type of substrate used. The result can be readily visualised or quantified using an ELISA reader.

1. Antibody adsorbed to plate

   wash

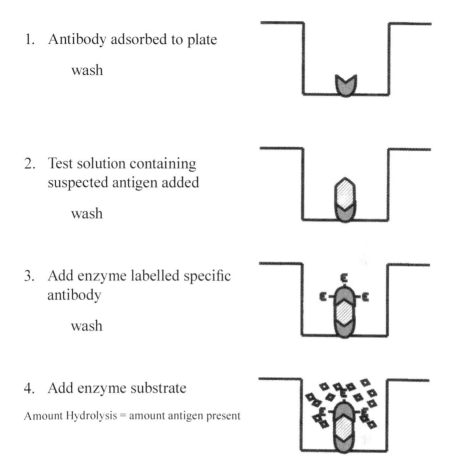

2. Test solution containing suspected antigen added

   wash

3. Add enzyme labelled specific antibody

   wash

4. Add enzyme substrate

Amount Hydrolysis = amount antigen present

Fig. 7.15 The Direct ELISA for detecting antigen

Indirect:

This is also referred to as double sandwich for antigen detection.

1. Coat the plate with 100µl of the capture antibody.
2. Wash three times with 300ul per well of washing buffer and allow to dry.
3. Block with 100ul of the blocking buffer and keep overnight at 4°C or at 37⁰C for 2 hours. This will block any non-specific binding site on the surface of the antibody. The blocking agent is the concentrated solution of a non-interacting protein BSA or casein which blocks non-specific absorptions of other proteins to the plate.

4. Add the antigen-containing sample to plate and incubate for 2 hours at 37°C. Wash three times to remove any unbound antigen.
5. Add the second antiviral antibody, this is the detecting antibody and incubate for 2 hours at 37°C. Wash three times to remove any unbound antibody.
6. Add the enzyme labelled (anti immunoglobulin secondary antibody) and incubate for 1 hour at 37°C. The secondary antibody binds to the detecting antibody.
7. Add the substrate and incubate in the dark at room temperature. Observe the colour change and stop the reaction with H_2SO_4 or 3M NaOH.

Antibody Detection by ELISA

The use of ELISA for the detection of anti viral antibodies have been widely used for HIV, hepatitis, yellow fever, measles, mumps, rubella and a host of other important viral diseases. The purpose of antibody detection can both be qualitative in which case the test provides a simple negative or positive results, or it can be quantitative to determine the antibody titre. Antibody detection by ELISA test can also be direct or indirect.

Direct
Procedure
1. Coat the ELISA plate with 100ul of a known antigen.
2. Add 100ul of the sample (usually patient serum) and incubate at 37°C for 2 hours. Wash three times to remove unbound antibody.
3. Add enzymes–labelled species specific anti immuno-lobulin and incubate again for 2 hours at 37°C. Wash to remove excess enzyme.
4. Add the 100ul of substrate and incubate for about 20-30 minutes in the dark at room temperature.
5. When the colour develops, stop the reaction with H_2SO_4 and read the test visually or using ELISA reader.

1. Antibody adsorbed to plate

    wash

2. Test solution containing
    suspected antigen added

    wash

3. Add enzyme labelled specific
    antibody

    wash

4. Add enzyme substrate

Amount Hydrolysis = amount antigen present

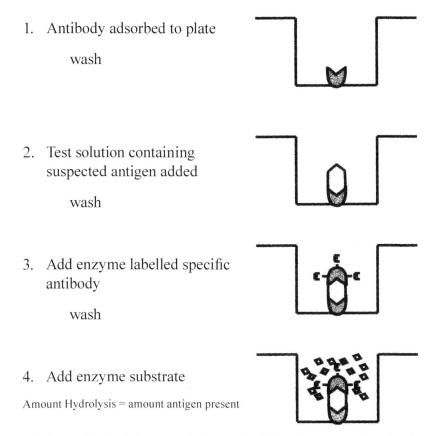

Fig. 7.16. The Direct ELISA method for the assay of antibody

Indirect (IgM Capture ELISA)

Procedure

1. Coat the plate with the capture antibody diluted in dilution buffer and incubate at 4°C overnight. The capture antibody is usually a species specific anti IgM immunoglobulin prepared in the animal species whose serum is to be tested.

2. Add the test serum (human serum) in PBS-Tween 20 and incubate at 37oC for 2 hours.

3. Add the known antigen diluted in PBS-Tween 20 and incubate at 37°C for 2 hours. Wash to remove unbound antigen. Known specific enzyme labelled antigen can be added at this stage instead of the antigen alone.

4. Wash plate and add the enzyme-labelled anti-species specific antiserum to the virus diluted in PBS-Tween 20 and again incubate at 37°C for 2 hours. This stage should be ommitted if the second option in step 3 was done. See Fig. 13.3

5. Wash, and then add the substrate. Incubate in the dark at room temperature for 30 minutes. Observe the colour change and stop the reaction with H_2SO_4

Visually read the test or use an ELISA reader. Determine the OD value, or visually observe the colour intensity. The colour change is proportional to the amount of virus specific IgM in the serum tested. A good control which includes a known negative, weak and strong positive sera must be included.

1. Anti-IgM adsorbed to plate

    wash

2. Test serum sample added

    wash

1. Reference viral solution

Reference enzyme labeled viral antigen solution added

Reference enzyme labeled virus specific antiserum added

Enzyme substrate Added

Mount hydrolysed

Anti IgM antibody in the sample

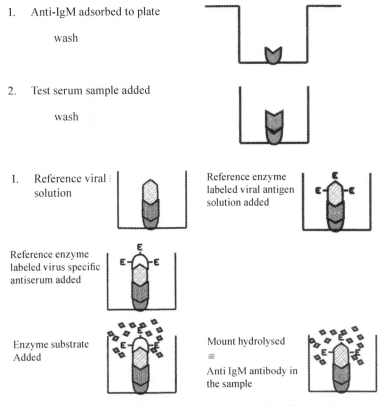

Fig. 7.17: The double Antibody sandwich ELISA
for measuring antibody (IgM ELISA)

Competitive ELISA

In the competitive ELISA, either an antigen or an antibody is bound to the solid phase surface. The labelled antigen competes for primary antibody binding sites with the unlabelled (unknown) sample antigen. The more antigen in the unknown sample, the less labelled antigen is retained in the well and the weaker the signal. A measured amount of the enzyme labelled component is added with the patient's serum. The labelled component competes with the unlabelled component in the patient's serum for binding to the component in the solid phase. The solid phase is then exposed to the substrate.

If the test sample contains a large component against the solid phase, it will bind almost all the sites in the component in the solid phase leaving little or nothing for the enzyme –labelled antigen or antibody to bind. The result of such is that there will be little or no colour change. If the test sample contains very little component against the solid phase component, the labelled antigen or antibody will bind almost all and the colour intensity will be more.

In contrast with the non-competitive ELISA, absence of colour is interpreted as positive while presence of colour change indicates that the sample is negative. The procedure is as follows:

Procedure
1. Coat the plate with 100ul of known antigen and incubate overnight at 4oC.
2. Add 100ul of the patient's serum and the enzyme-labelled antibody. Incubate at 37°C for 2 hours. The patient's antibody competes with the enzyme labelled antibodies for binding the antigen. Wash three times to remove unbound serum.
3. Add 100ul of the substrate and incubate for 30 minutes.
4. Observe absence or presence of colour change. Little or no colour means that the test sample is positive for the antibody while a colour of high intensity signifies a negative antibody result.

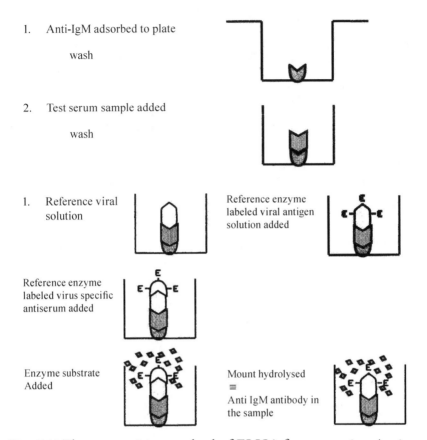

1. Anti-IgM adsorbed to plate

   wash

2. Test serum sample added

   wash

1. Reference viral solution

Reference enzyme labeled viral antigen solution added

Reference enzyme labeled virus specific antiserum added

Enzyme substrate Added

Mount hydrolysed
≡
Anti IgM antibody in the sample

Fig. 7.18.The competitive method of ELISA for measuring Antigen

Western Blot

The Western Blot (WB), often times called Immunoblot, is a serological test used to detect specific proteins in tissue homogenates, sera or extracts. It uses gel electrophoresis to separate proteins according to their molecular weights either by length of their polypeptides or by the 3-D structure of the proteins. When proteins are denatured and put into an electric field, they will all move towards the positive pole at the same rate, with no separation by size. An environment that allows different sized proteins to move at different rates is provided by polyacrylamide, a polymer of acrylamide monomers. When this polymer is formed, it turns into a gel through which the proteins can pass easily with the help of electrical voltage. This process is known as polyacrylamide gel electrophoresis (PAGE). A polyacrylamide gel is not solid but is made of a laberynth of tunnels through a meshwork of fibers. The separated proteins, which in this case may be a virus or its antigen, can now be transferred into nitrocellulose strips where they can be detected using specific antibodies to the antigens. The use of monoclonal antibodies readily comes to mind here. Monoclonal or polyclonal antibodies are available for many proteins or viral antigens.

Reagents
1.Resolving gel pH 8.8)
The resolving gel is prepared as shown below, depending on the concentration. The concentration of acrylamide determines the resolution of the gel. The greater the concentration of the acrylamide, the better the resolution of small molecular weight proteins whereas the lower the concentration, the better the resolution of the higher molecular weight proteins.

Percentage of gel	8%	10%	12.5%
30: 0.8% w/v acrylamide:bisacrylamide	2ml	2.5ml	3.1ml
1.0M Tris-Cl pH 8.8	3ml	3ml	3ml
20% SDS	38ul	38ul	38ul
dH$_2$O	2.43ml	1.9ml	1.3ml
Mix together. Add APS and TEMED just before pouring			
10% APS	36ul	36ul	36ul
TEMED	5ul	5ul	5ul
	7.5ml	7.5ml	7.5ml

Table 7.3 Preparation of resolving gel

2. Stacking gel(pH 6.8)
Use 4% stack for <10% resolving. gel and 6% stack for >10% gel.

Percentage of stack	4%	6%
30:0.8% w/v acryl:bisacryl	660 ul	1ml
1M Tris-Cl pH6.8	630 ul	630 ul
20% SDS	25 ul	25 ul
dH$_2$O	3.6 ml	3.6 ml
Mix together. Add APS and TEMED just before pouring		
10% APS	25ul	25ul
TEMED	5ul	5ul
	5ml	5ml

Table 7.4 Preparation of stacking gel

3. Sample loading buffer (Laemmli loading dye) 3X stock:

1M Tris-Cl pH 6.8 2.4 ml

20% SDS 3 ml

Glycerol (100%) 3 ml

B-mercaptoethanol 1.6 ml

Bromophenol blue 0.006g

10 ml (store 4°C)

(i)   Protein samples are prepared in 1X sample loading buffer (also called Laemmli dye)

(ii) To 6 ul protein sample, add 3 ul 3X Laemmli dye stock.

(iii) Boil 3 minutes before loading gel.

4. 10X Running buffer (also called Laemmli buffer):

This is prepared as shown

Tris base   30.3 g

Glycine   144 g

SDS   10 g

Make to 1L with dH_2O

For example, to make a 500 ml 1X buffer, dilute 50 ml 10X stock with 450 ml dH20.

Gel should be run at room temperature for about 1 hour at a constant voltage of 200V until the bromophenol blue dye is just off.

Materials

Gel plates

Buffer chambers

Comb

Power pack

Procedure

1.   Set up gel plates before mixing the gels.

2.   Use the thin spacers and choose a comb number corresponding to the numbers of desired wells.

3.   Make both resolving gel and stack without APS or TEMED.

4. Mix and pour about 3-3.5ml per gel plate. Before it polymerises, add APS and TEMED to the stack mix and pour it gently on top of the resolving gel.
5. Put in the comb and allow between 15-20 minutes to solidify.
6. Gels can be kept overnight at 4°C if well wrapped to prevent drying out and if the comb is kept in too.
7. Wash out wells with distilled water to remove unpolymerised acrylamide before loading.

Running of Gel
Procedure
1. Clamp in your gel and fill both buffer chambers with gel running buffer,
2. Pipet about 5µg of the sample into the gel adjusting the volume according to the amount of protein in your sample.
3. Include a lane with molecular weight markers.
4. Attach the power leads and run the gel until the blue dye front reaches the bottom.
5. Run at between 200- 250 constant voltage. This may take between 50-60 minutes depending on the thickness of the gel. You may need to adjust to the thickness of the gel.
6. Remove the gel from the power supply and process further.
7. Visualise your proteins using Coomassie Brilliant Blue, Silver stain, or any of the other protein stains.

Transfer into Nitrocellulose strips
In order to make the separated proteins or antigens accessible to antibodies, they must be transferred onto a nitrocellulose membrane.
Procedure
1. Place the membrane on top of the gel and place a stack of tissue paper on top.
2. Place the entire stack in a buffer solution. The buffer will move by capillary action through the paper carrying along

with it the proteins. The proteins will move from the gel into the nitrocellulose membrane without distrupting their organisational structures from the gel.

Blocking and Detection

Procedure

1. Place the membrane in a dilution of protein usually BSA or non fat milk to which a small percentage of Tween 20 has been added to bind to any remaining sticky places on the nitrocellulose.
2. Add about 0.5-5ug test antibody and incubate at 37^0C for 1-2hrs or at 4^0C overnight.
3. Rinse the membranes to remove any unbound antibodies
4. Add the secondary antibody i.e. species specific antibody -conjugated enzyme (Horseradish peroxidase) to the membrane. This will bind to its specific protein.
5. Add the appropriate substrate and incubate in the dark for about 30-45 minutes. Colour bands will be formed where the antibodies have bound with the specific proteins. This can be visualised using the chemiluscent lamp or it can be photographed.

The confirmatory test for HIV uses the Western Blot technique to detect HIV specific proteins.(See Fig. 18.1)

Neutralisation Assay for the Identification of Viruses

Neutralisation assay is considered to be the standard against which other serologic methods are measured. It measures the ability of antibodies to block viral infectivity and therefore it also correlates with protection from infection. Although neutralisation assay is rarely used as a diagnostic tool because it is time consuming, the method still finds its application in the final identification and classification of viruses as it is the gold standard for final confirmation of new viral isolates. Prior to the performance of neutralisation test, it is very important to determine the number of viral particles in the suspension stock. The number of viral particles present in clinical specimens depends to a large extend on the nature and property of the virus, the organ or tissue infected, and the concentration of the virus in the specimen. The process of determining the number of infectious virions in a virus stock is called titration. This is done by calculating the 50% end point in the appropriate indicator medium (tissue culture, embryonated egg, albino mice etc).

Determination of 50% End Point

Viruses only grow in living tissues e.g. tissue culture, embryonated eggs or laboratory animals, where they produce cytopathic effects, death or paralysis. Therefore, estimation of live or infectious virus particles in a virus suspension is made by estimating visible effects of a single particle in form of CPE, death or paralysis. This is done by calculating the infective titre. The infective titre is the proportionate distance between the dilution over 50% and dilution below 50% plus the dilution above 50%.

Titration of virus is done in the appropriate indicator system like tissue culture, mice or embryonated egg. If tissue culture is the indicator system, this can be seeded into 96 well microtitre plates or tubes.

Virus titration starts with the making of fold dilutions of the viral suspension. This is usually a 10-fold dilution starting from 1:10. The procedure is shown below (Fig. 7.19).

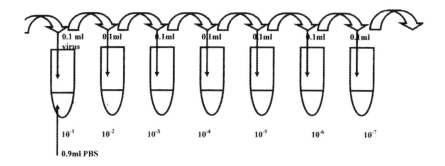

Fig 7.19 Serial 10-fold dilution of virus suspension

Procedure

1. Make a 10 fold serial dilution of the virus suspension starting from 10^{-1} to 10^{-7} (see diagram).
2. Select seven sterile dilution or Khan tubes. Using a sterile pipette, put 0.9ml of PBS into each of the tubes.
3. Using a 1 ml pipette or pipettor with ART tips, add 0.1ml of the virus suspension into the first tube. Mix thoroughly. Remove 0.1 ml of the mixed suspension and add into the second tube. Discard the pipette or tip. Use a new pipette or tip to remove 0.1 ml suspension into the next tube. Continue this procedure unto the last tube. Discard 0.1ml from the last tube.
4. Starting from the highest dilution i.e 10^{-7}, inoculate a given volume e.g 0.2ml into each of six wells of confluent monolayer of susceptible cell in the 96-well plate.
5. Add 2% MEM or any other medium to make up the volume in the well. Leave about 6 wells uninoculated to serve as control.
6. Incubate at 37oC and check for virus cytopathic effect daily. Record the number of cells showing CPE per day. Terminate the reading when the uninoculated control wells begin to show degeneration.
7. Calculate the dilution that causes CPE in 50% of the wells by the method of Reed and Muench. This will give you the titre of the virus which is measured in tissue culture infective dose (TCID).

Calculation of TCID$_{50}$ (Reed and Muench)

Not all virus particles are infective. The titration method only recognises the infected particle. If, for example, only 1 unit of infectious virus is introduced into a susceptible tissue culture, the cell will be killed, but this 1 unit is randomly distributed somewhere in the suspension. When this suspension is diluted to contain that 1 unit in half of the ml, the suspension is said to contain 1TCID$_{50}$ per inoculated dose.

This is calculated using the inoculation result (4-7) above as shown below.

Virus dilution (a)	Mortality ratio (b)	Died (c)	Survived (d)	Accumulated values			
				Died (e)	Survived (f)	Ratio (g)	Percentage (%) (h)
10^{-1}	6/6	6	0	22	0	22/22	100
10^{-2}	6/6	6	0	16	0	16/16	100
10^{-3}	4/6	4	2	10	2	10/12	83
10^{-4}	3/6	3	3	6	5	6/11	54
10^{-5}	2/6	2	4	3	9	3/12	25
10^{-6}	1/6	1	5	1	14	1/15	6.6
10^{-7}	0/6	0	6	0	20	0/20	0

Table 7.5 Mortality and survival pattern of inoculated laboratory animal

The end point is the dilution at which a certain populaton of the test indicator shows reaction. The most accurate and desirable is that proportion in which ½ of the test sample reacts. Accumulated values for the total number that died or survived are obtained by adding in the direction of the arrows. The accumulated mortality ratio (g) is equal to the accumulated number of dead animals over accumulated total number inoculated (e+f). The mortality in 10^{-4} dilution is higher than 50% and at 10^{-5} dilution, it is lower than 50%. The proportionate distance (PD) of the 50% mortality end point lies within these two dilutions.

PD = % mortality at dilution immediately above 50% - 50 / % mortality at dilution immediately above 50% - mortality at dilution below 50%.

Substituting $\dfrac{54-50}{54-25} = \dfrac{4}{29} = 0.14$

Logarithmically, the distance between any dilution is a function of incremental step used (e.g 2-fold, 4-fold, 5-fold or 10-fold). The PD must be corrected by the dilution factor which in the example above is 1.The titre of the viral suspension is the log of dilution above 50% plus the PD multiplied by 1. In the example above, therefore, the $TCID_{50}$ is $Log_{10}10^{-4.14}$. Since titers are the reciprocal of their dilutions, the titer of the above virus suspension is $log10^{4.14}/$ 0.2ml.

Interpretation
At $10^{4.14}$ the viral unit in the suspension is 1 Unit per 0.2ml
  $10^{3.14} = 10$ units   0.2 ml
  $10^{2.14}=100$ units/0.2ml
$10^{1.14}=1000$ units/0.2ml
Undiluted=10000 units/0.2ml

This can be adjusted to whatever desired concentration and volume.

Calculation of Titre by Karber Formula
Titres can also be calculated using the Karber formula shown below:
$Log\ TCID_{50} = L-d(S-0.5)$ where:
L = log of lowest dilution in the test showing 100% CPE
d = difference between log dilution steps.(This is always 1 for a 10-fold dilution).
S = sum of proportion of positive tests showing CPE
Substituting from the example above:
L = -2; d= 1.0; S=(1+0.83+0.54+0.25+0.066 – 0.5)
  = - 2 – 1(2.686-0.5) which equals – 2 - 2.186 = - 4.19
Virus titre = $Log\ TCID_{50}$ = -4.19/0.2ml and $10^{4.83}\ TCID_{50}/ml$

How to calculate exact 100 $TCID_{50}$ from titre
From the example above, 100 units of the virus is located between the $10^{2.14}$ and $10^{3.14}$. Therefore, to capture the exact dilution with the $100TCID_{50}$, make a serial dilution from the original viral dilution to 10^2. Look for the log of 0.14 and subtract the sum from 1. The Log of 0.14 is equal to -0.85.

1- 0.85= 0.15.

Take 0.15 part of the 10^2 of the virus suspension into 0.85 part of diluent. That dilution contains the 100TCID$_{50}$.

Alternatively, the exact 100TCID$_{50}$ can also be calculated as shown below:

From the stock virus titre of $10^{4.83}$ TCID$_{50}$/ml, the virus dilution of $10^{-4.83}$ gives the 1TCID$_{50}$, 100TCID$_{50}$ = $10^{-2.83}$.

To make this dilution from virus stock of $10^{4.83}$ TCID50/ml

First prepare $10^{-0.83}$ virus dilution thus: $10^{-0.83}$ = $1/10^{0.83}$ = $1/6.76$ (where 6.76 = antilog of 0.83), Take 1 part of the virus stock plus 5.76 parts diluent.

3. Again take 1 part of this dilution plus 9 parts diluents.

This will give a dilution of = $10^{-1.83}$.

4.   Take 1 part of the $10^{-1.83}$ dilution and add 9 parts of diluent = $10^{-2.83}$ as the 100TCID$_{50}$.

5.   This will give a final dilution of $10^{-2.83}$ which contains the 100 TCID$_{50}$.

Neutralisation Test in Tissue Culture

There are usually two methods of neutralisation test. The Beta method which uses the constant virus, varying serum technique and the Alpha method which uses the constant serum varying virus. The Beta method measures the neutralisation end point. The Beta method is preferred in most laboratories. The Alpha method is used when there is no physical access to the serum. This method is used for antiviral assays or when the effect of a reagent or chemical against any virus is to be determined. The Alpha method determines the neutralisation index (NI).

Materials
96 –well tissue culture plates
The desired cell line
Medium
1,2,5 or 10 ml pipettes
Pipettors with ART tips

Beta Neutralistion Test

Procedure

1. Calculate the titre of your virus as described above by the method of Reed and Muench or Karber method.

2. Make two fold serial dilution of the known +ve specific serum or test serum starting from either 1:2 or 1:10.

3. Calculate from the titre of the virus the dilution that contains 100TCID50 per dilution. This is the constant virus and it is the working dilution (WD).

4. Add equal volume of the known specific positive serum or test serum to equal volume of the WD.

5. Incubate mixture at 37°C for one hour for antibody antigen reaction.

6. Two options are opened at this point: (a) Inoculate twice the volume of the virus/serum mixture into an already confluent cell line in the tissue culture plates and allow to absorb for 1-2 hours at 37°C. (b) Add wet a known volume containing a calculated number of freshly trypsinised cells into the virus antiserum mixture.

7. Whichever option, incubate the inoculated plates at 37°C and check for viral CPE daily.

8. For virus control, make a serial ten fold dilution of the WD from 10^{-1} to 10^{-4}. Inoculate each dilution into four replicate wells/tubes of cell.

9. Incubate both test and control wells/tubes at 37°C and check daily for inhibition of CPE. The final test result can be read when the virus control well/tubes show complete CPE.

The complete inhibition of the 100 $TCID_{50}$ of the virus by the known type-specific antiserum is regarded as positive and indicative of the viral agent. Apart from using this test to identif a virus, NT can also be used to determine the titre of serum to determine previous exposure. In this case, the titre of the serum is the highest dilution that completely inhibits the appearance of viral CPE. High titre of serum identifies the virus and previous exposure to such virus.

Plaque Assay

Virus can also be quantitated by the plaque formation technique. A known volume of virus suspension is inoculated into cell culture and overlayed with an agar or cellulose overlay. Because the spread of the virus is restricted by the overlay, each viral particle grows and forms an area of necrotic plaque. This plaque represents one viral unit and its progeny. Since each plaque represents the progeny of the virus causing the plaque, plaque is often used to purify viruses. Quantitation by the plaque method is as follows:

Materials
Agar, Agarose or Methyl cellulose
Cells
6,12, or 24 well tissue culture plates or plastic tissue
culture flasks
Medium
1, 2, 5 or 10ml pipettes
Pipettor with ART tips
Stain (Methyl blue, Neutral red, crystal violet etc)

Procedure
1. Prepare methyl cellulose (or any other agar medium). Concentration can range between 0.8% to 1.5%.
2. Grow the cells in the appropriate flask, bottles or plates, and allow to become confluent.
3. Make a serial 10-fold dilution of the viral suspension starting from 10^{-1} - 10^{6}.
4. Inoculate between 0.1 – 0.2 ml of each dilution into about 4 wells. Spread the inoculum all over the surface to prevent dehydration and for equal spread of the inoculum over the cells.
5. Incubate at 37°C for 1 hour in an atmosphere of 5% CO_2.
6. Add 1% methyl cellulose overlay medium. The volume of methyl cellulose overlay will depend on the type of

container used. For 24 well plate- 1 ml, and for 6 well plate – 5ml.

7. After 3-4 days aspirate the overlay medium completely.
8. Fix and stain the infected monolayer with 0.5-2ml of a mixture containing 5% formalin and 1.3% crystal violet. Staining should take between 20-30 minutes.
9. Rinse the plate thoroughly under tap water.
10. You can now count the number of plaques formed per dilution.

The sizes or forms of plaque may vary according to the virus. The number of the plaques formed can be calculated and recorded as plaque forming unit per ml.

11. In the example shown in Fig. 7.22, the plaque titre of the virus is 10×10^{-6} PFU/0.2ml or 1×10^{-7} PFU/0.2ml.

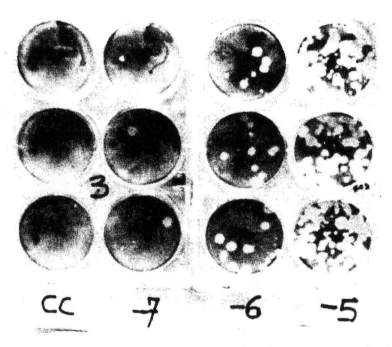

Fig 7.20 Quantitation of poliovirus by the plaque assay method in HEp-2C cell monolayer

Neutralisation by Plaque Reduction Neutralization Test (PRNT)

The plaque reduction neutralization test(PRNT) is more sensitive and more accurate than the standard NT test. To perform the PRNT the following steps are taken:

Infectivity titre of stock virus is determined by inoculating 10-fold serial dilution to 6-wells of each row of 24-well plate. The wells are then overlayed with semi-solid or solid overlay medium. Cells are incubated at the appropriate temperature (35-37°C) and observed for 3-5 days. The cells are then stained as described above to determine plaque counts.

A working dilution (WD) containing between 20-50 plaque forming units (PFU) per 0.1ml is determined.

Equal amount of the WD is mixed with type specific known antiserum and allowed alongside with the virus dilution to stand for 1 hour at 37°C or at room temperature.

Afterwards,0.2ml of the serum-virus dilutions and 0.1ml virus control are inoculated into triplicate wells of the 24-well plate. Additional 0.1 ml MEM is added to virus control wells.

The plates are then incubated at 37°C in an atmosphere of 5% CO_2 for 1 hour for virus absorption.

During the incubation, the semi-solid overlay is prewarmed to 45°C and 1ml of the medium is gently overlayed on the cells.

The inoculated cells are covered and incubated at 37°C at 5% CO_2 for 2-7 days.

After 2-7, days depending on the nature of the virus, aspirate the overlay. Fix and stain as described above.

Count the visible plaques in both the serum-virus mixtures wells and the virus control wells.

An 80% or greater plaque reduction in the serum -virus wells, compared with the control wells is regarded as positive and confirms the identity of the virus.

Determination of Antiviral Activity by Plaque Reduction Neutralisation Test

The Plaque Reduction Neutralisation Test is a very good test for determining the antiviral activities of antiviral agents. This principle is based on the ability of the antiviral drug when mixed with the virus to reduce the number of plaques by about 80% or greater when compared with the virus alone.

Since viruses have different sensitivities to different cells, this result may be influenced by the type of cells used. The result can also be influenced by the concentration of the virus and the time between virus inoculation and harvest. It is therefore necessary, before performing the test, to determine in the cell of choice the toxic dose of the drug. The procedure is as follows:

Materials
Antiviral agent
Plastic plates
Medium
Piettes and pipettors
ART tips

Procedure
1. Determine the toxic dose of the antiviral agent in the cell of choice.
2. Determine the plaque titre of the virus in plaque forming unit.
3. Make a serial dilution of the antiviral drug starting from the minimum toxic dose.
4. After step 3, two separate steps can be taken.
   (a) Mix equal volume of the virus with the different concentrations of the drug and incubate at 37°C for 1 hour. Incubate the virus suspension containing the challenge dose under the same condition.
   (b) Inoculate 0.2ml of the virus-drug mixture and 0.1ml of the virus control into duplicate wells in the 24-well plate and incubate at 37°C at 5% CO_2 for 1 hour.

Inoculate equal amount of the challenge virus suspension into four duplicate wells in the 24-well plate and allow for 1 hour of absorption at 37°C. Add equal amount of different dilutions of the antiviral agent to the overlay medium and mix very well.

Overlay the infected cells with 0.1 ml of the overlay containing the antiviral drug.

5. Incubate all plates at 37°C in an atmosphere of 5% CO_2.

6. Cells can be checked after 5-7 days for plaque. Fix and stain the cells as already described. Count the number of plaques per concentration. A reduction of 80% and greater between the observed number of plaques in the control and the infected cells is regarded as positive.

The Alpha method of neutralisation test in cell culture can also be used, in which case, the neutralisation index, which is the difference between the titre of challenge virus alone minus the titre of virus in the virus-drug mixture, is recorded. neutralisation index greater than 1 and above is regarded as positive antiviral activity against the virus.

Further Reading

Chromaitree T. Baldwin CD and H. Lucia. "Role of the Virology Lab in Diagnosis and Management of Patients with Central Nervous System Disease". *Clin Microbiol Review*, 1989 2(1) 1-14.

Fundenberg HH, Stites DP, Caldwell JL and Wells JV. *Basic and Clinical Immunolog*. Lang Medical Publications 1976.

Gardener PS, Grandieu M, and McQuillan J. Comparison of Immunoflourescence and Immunoperoxidise Methods for Viral Dignosis at a Distance". A WHO collaborative study. Bull WHO 56, 105, 1978.

Gardner PS, McQuillin J. Rapid. *Virus diagnosis: application of immunoflourescence*. Toronto: Bulterworth and Co Ltd 1974.

Gregory A Storch. *Essentials of Diagnostic Virology*. Churchill Livingstone, New York, 2000.

Hsiung GD, Caroline KY, Fong and Marie L. Landry. Hsiung's Diagnostic Virology 4th ed. Yale University Press 1994.

John R Stephenson, Allan Warnes. *Diagnostic Virology Protocols.* Humama Press 2007

Lyerla HC and Forrester FT. "Immunoflourescence Methods in Virology". Washington DC. US Dept of HEW, Public Health Service, 1979.

Mary L. Christiensen. *Basic Laboratory Procedures in Diagnostic Virology.* Charles C. Thomas Publishers Ltd 1977.

Voller A, Bidwell DE and Barlett A. The Enzyme Linked Immunosobent Essay (ELISA). *A guide with abstracts of microplate application.* Dynatech Europe, Borough House, Reu du Pre, Guernsey, Great Britain. 1979.

WHO. Polio Laboratory Manual, 4th ed. "Immunisation, Vaccines and Biologicals."World Health Organization CH-1211, Geneva Switzerland. 2004.

Laemmli, U. K. (1970). "Cleavage of Structural Proteins during the Assembly of the Head of Bacteriophage T4. *Nature* 227, 680-685.

CHAPTER 8

THE POLYMERASE CHAIN REACTION (PCR)

The Polymerase Chain Reaction (PCR) is a simple yet very complex molecular biological procedure with a tremendous power and versatility for DNA manipulation and analysis. The PCR has revolutionised the approach to molecular biology and medical research. The procedure is predicated on the presence of some reactants, some of which are present at very low initial concentration but which increases dramatically as the reaction proceeds. Example of this is the DNA template. Others are present at concentrations that hardly change during the reactions. To this group are the deoxynucleotides (dNTPs) and the primers.

The PCR works in three distinct steps that are governed by temperature viz-

1. The template DNA is denatured to separate the complementary strands.

2. The reaction is cooled to an annealing temperature to allow the oligonucleotide primers hybridise to the DNA template.

3. Finally the reaction is heated to a temperature close to optimal polymerisation temperature for polymerase. These procedures result in the production of microgram quantities of DNA from picogram of the starting materials. The PCR allows the amplification of the target

sequences of the DNA almost 100,000 fold after about 30-35 cycles in two hours.

The principle of the PCR is based on the amplification of the DNA segment between two regions of a known sequence. Two oligonucleotide primers usually derived from the desired segment of the DNA to be amplified are used as primers. These two primers, the forward and the reverse, have different sequences and are complementary to the sequences on the opposite strands of the DNA template.

The Basics Ingredients of PCR
The basic ingredients of the PCR amplification are:
1. The target dsDNA usually referred to as the template. This could be the direct DNA or a cDNA transcribed from the RNA by reverse transcription.
2. Two Primers – short oligonucleotides. They act as sites for initiation by the DNA polymerase. It defines the area of the template to be copied.
3. Taq Polymerase is a 9.4 kDa protein that has two catalytic activities. The enzyme is thermostable and has a half life of around 40 minutes at 95°C. This is equivalent to about 50 cycles under standard PCR conditions. The Taq polymerase is a good general purpose enzyme that is capable of amplifying products up to 2-4 kbp efficiently.
4. Nucleotides. These are the building blocks and are present in the form of the four deoxynucleotides (dATP, dGTP, dCTP and dTTP). The primer is extended during amplification in the presence of dNTPs.
5. PCR buffers. These include:
100 mM Tris-HCl
500mM KCl
15mM MgCl2
0.1% Tween-20
0.1% NP-40
1 Mg ml^{-1} gelatin

As stated above, the PCR is temperature dependent and involves 3 distinct steps.

1. The first step is the denaturation stage of 94°C. The double stranded DNA melts open to single stranded DNA. At this point, enzymatic reactions stop.
2. Annealing. This is achieved at temperature 42-54°C. Hydrogen bonds form between the single stranded primer and template, the polymerase attaches to the duplex and starts to copy the template.
3. Extension. This is usually at 72°C. Bases complementary are coupled to the primer on the 3' end. Usually the DNA polymerase synthesises a new DNA strand complementary to the DNA template by adding dNTPs that are complementary to the template in the 5' to 3' direction condensing the 5'- phosphate group of the dNTPs with the 3' -hydroxyl group.

PCR Protocol
Equipment needed
Ice bucket
Micro centrifuge
Micro centrifuge PCR tube
Thermal cycler
Gel electrophoresis

Materials and Reagents
Thermostable DNA polymerase (Taq DNA polymerase)
2 mM dNTPs
Oligonucleotide primers
Template DNA
Mineral Oil (optional)
0.8% agarose
50 x TAE

Protocol:

1.   **RNA extraction**

For RNA viruses the RNA must first be reverse transcribed to obtain the complementary DNA (cDNA) which provides the DNA template for amplification. Therefore, the RNA must be extracted from the virus lysate. RNA is extracted by phenol extraction. However, there are some commercial extraction kits, the most common is the Qiagen RNA extraction kit.

Materials
Buffer AVE
Buffer AVL
Buffer AW1, AW2 and carrier RNA
1.5ml microcentrifuge.
Ethanol (96-100%)
2ml Collection tube
Microcentrifuge

Procedure
The RNA extraction and RT-PCR described here is as practiced by the Respiratory and Enterovirus Branch of the Centers for Disease Control and Prevention, Atlanta Georgia, USA.

RNA Extraction

1. Pipette 560ul of AVL buffer into 1.5 ml eppendorf tube.
2. Add 140ul of cell culture virus harvest (or source of RNA).
3. Incubate at room temperature for 10 minutes.
4. Centrifuge the 1.5ml briefly to remove drops from side.
5. Add 560ul of ethanol to the sample and mix, pulse vortex for 15 seconds.
6. Again centrifuge briefly to remove drops from inside the lid.
7. Repeat step 6 with the remaining sample.
8. Carefully open the column and add 500 ml of buffer AW1. Close the cap and centrifuge at 6000x5 (8000rpm) for 1 minute. Place the column in a clean 2-ml collection tube provided and discard the tube containing the filterate.

9. Carefully open the column and add 500ml of buffer AW2. Close cap and centrifuge at full speed 20,000g (14,000 rpm) for 3 minutes. You may repeat this process again or go to step 10.

10. Place the QIAmp column in 1.5ml microcentrifuge. Discard the old collection. Carefully open and add 60 ul of buffer AVE equilibrated to room temperature. Close the cap and incubate at room temperature for 1 minute. Centrifuge at 8000 rpm for 1 minute.

11. Store the extracted RNA at -20^{0}C.

Reverse Transcriptase PCR (RT-PCR)

The reverse transcription PCR (RT-PCR) is performed on the extracted RNA as follows:

Mix I
Make Mix 1 solution in a 1.5ml PCR tube.

(1)	Primer 1	-	1 ul
	Primer 2	-	1 ul
	RNA	-	5 ul

Mix thoroughly and heat at 95 °C for 5 minutes. Place on ice while proceeding to the next stage.

Mix II
Make Mix II as follows:

| 10X PCR buffer - | 10 ul | - | Multiply by the number of reactions to be run. |

dNTPs (each) -	4 ul
RNAse -	1 ul
RT -	1 ul
Primers -	3 ul
Taq Polymerase -	1 ul

ETF/RNAse free Water - 73 ul.

1. Mix thoroughly by brief centrifugation and add 73 ul each of Mix II into the Mix I RNA tube. Mix thoroughly by centrifugation. The reaction is now ready for RT-PCR.

2. Place the tube in a thermal cycler and programme for the following temperatures.

42°C   for 60 minutes
94°C   for 5 minutes
94°C   for 1 minute
55°C   for 1 minute
72°C   for 1 minute
72°C   for 2 minutes
4°C   for ever

PCR temperature regimes can vary at the different steps. Individual must therefore establish the right temperature for their reactions. This can be easily done by selecting and creating the best programme in the thermal cycler.

3. After the required number of cycles, remove the tube from the thermal cycler.
4. Analyse between 5 and 15 ul of the PCR product on an agarose gel using the right molecular marker.

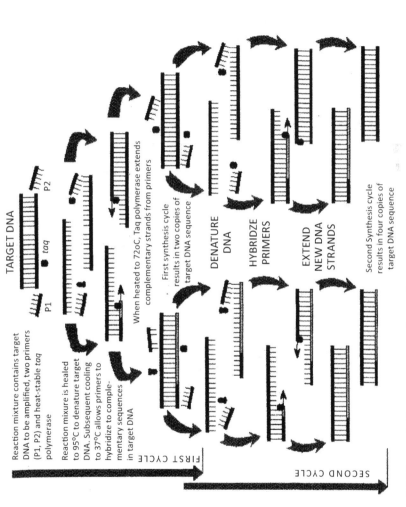

Fig. 8.1 DNA amplification using the Polymerase Chain Reaction Source: DNA Science

Gel Electrophoresis

After the PCR run, the PCR product (amplicon) must be checked to confirm if there is any PCR product and if the product is of the desired size. This is done by running the product through an agarose gel.

Gel electrophoresis is a procedure for separating a mixture of the charged molecules through a stationary material (gel) in an electrical field. The molecules are separated according to electrical charge, size and other physical properties.

Materials:
6 X Dye
Agarose
Ethidium bromide
1 X TBE

Equipment:
Gel electrophoresis tank
Transluminiscent UV lamp
Microwave oven

Procedures:
1. Weigh 800 ug (0.8gm) of agarose in 80 ml of 1 X TBE buffer and heat in the microwave oven for 3-5 minutes to melt.
2. Add 4.5 ul of Ethidium bromide and gently mix.
3. Remove the PCR product from the thermal cycler.
4. Pour the agarose into the gel plate and insert the gel comb. Allow to solidify.
5. Cut a clean paraffin wax paper and drop 10 ul of the 6 X dye according to the number of PCR products.
6. Add 50ml of the PCR product to the dye and mix very well.
7. Remove the comb from the molten agarose and gently fill each well with 60 ul of the PCR- product mix but fill the first well with 15 ul of the molecular marker.
8. Insert the gel in plate into the running buffer.

9. Connect to the source of power, being careful to connect the right polarity (black to black and red to red).
10. Run for 2 hours at 65 volts or 12 volt overnight.
11. Remove and photograph under the UV transluminiscent lamp to observe the bands.

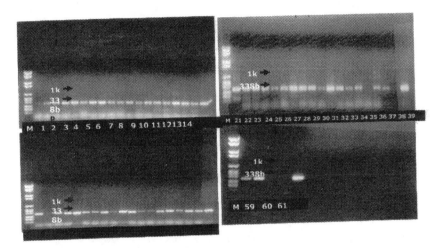

Fig.8.2 Gel eletrophoresis showing the sizes of PCR products.
Source: Oyero G.F. PhD Thesis, Department of Virology, College of Medicine, University of Ibadan, Nigeria.

The PCR products can be purified and later used for sequencing, cloning and diagnostic analysis. Cloning and sequencing is beyond the scope of this book.

The PCR has found wide application in virology. It has been widely used in the diagnosis of infections and other form of diseases and for the direct detection of infectious disease agents in clinical specimens. PCR has been very useful in the determination of viral load in HIV diagnosis and management of HIV infectivity. PCR has lately been widely used in the understanding of molecular epidemiology of diseases because of the process of sequencing and genotyping that can be derived from the PCR products. With the use of PCR, variations and mutation in genes can be detected easily.

The Real-Time PCR

The Real Time PCR also known as quantitative real time PCR (qPCR) as the name implies is a modification of the standard PCR that is used to monitor the progress of the PCR reaction in real time. The technique does not only monitor, but will also simultaneously quantify the PCR product after each cycle of the PCR amplification.

The Real Time PCR is based on the detection of a fluorescent produced by a reporter molecule which increases as the reaction proceeds. The fluorescence emitted by the reporter molecule manifolds as the PCR product accumulates with each cycle. It enables both detection and quantification of a specific sequence in a DNA sample. Based on the molecule used for detection, the real time PCR techniques can be categorised into two:

(1) Non-specific detection using DNA binding dyes and

(2) Specific detection which uses target specific probes.

In the non-specific detection, DNA binding dyes are used as fluorescence reporters to monitor the real time PCR as the product accumulates with each successive cycle of amplification. By recording the amount of fluorescence emission at each cycle, it is possible to monitor the PCR reaction during the exponential phase. A graph drawn between the log of the starting amount of template and the corresponding increase in the fluorescence of the dye fluorescence during the real time PCR will produce a linear relationship.

The SYBR^R Green is the most widely used ds DNA specific dye.

One disadvantage of the non-specific detection with the DNA binding dye is that the SYBR Green will also bind other dsDNA PCR products which may result in potential interference with or prevention of accurate quantification of the target.

In the specific detection using target specific probes, the real time PCR is done with oligonucleotide probes labelled with both reporter fluorescence dye and a quencher dye. This is the most accurate and reliable method. It uses a sequence – specific RNA or DNA based probe to quantify only the DNA containing the probe sequence. It therefore allows quantification only of the specific DNA. Because of this particular peculiarity of this method, it is possible to multiplex the reactions by using specific probes with different coloured labels. In this procedure, the PCR is prepared as usual. The reporter probe is added. During annealing, both probe and primers anneal to the DNA target.Polymerisation of new DNA strand is initiated from the primers; the polymerase degrades the probe thereby physically separating the florescent reporter from the quencher resulting in an increase in fluorescence.

Fluorescence is detected and measured in real time PCR thermocycler. The geometric increase corresponding to exponential increase of the product is used to determine the threshold cycle (Ct) in each reaction.

The relative concentration of DNA present during exponential phase of the reaction are determined by plotting fluorescence against cycle numbers on a logarithm scale. A threshold for detection of fluorescence above the background is determined. The cycle at which the fluorescence from a sample crosses the threshold is called the cycle threshold CT. Since the quantity of DNA doubles every cycle during exponential phase, relative amount of DNA can be calculated.

The introduction of real time PCR assay has led to significant improvements in the diagnosis of viral diseases. For example, the real time PCR has been able to shorten the period of wild polio detection by about 50-60%. This is because there is no need for post PCR processing such as pouring and cleaning of gels which is usually required for the standard PCR. The real time PCR is able to detect individual viruses in a mixture, and does not need to be separated before the test is run. Also in polio diagnosis, the real time PCR is able to directly detect circulating vaccine derived poliovirus (cVDPV) from the normal Sabin viruses without having to recur to the ELI.SA.

Below is a typical example of a real-time polymerase chain reaction of Sabin polio virus:

Materials
The reagents are normally supplied in a kit that contains the followings:

i. Primers and probes in Buffer A (Theses are the different poliovirus primer sets)
ii. Buffer B
iii. DTT
iv. Enzymes- (Roche Applied Science)
RNase Inhibitor
Reverse Transcriptase (RT)
Taq DNA Polymerase

Procedure
Extract RNA or use tissue culture isolate.
Make up the right mix for each primer set, i.e. Sabin, Pan Polio, Pan Entero and Serotypes.
Make up solution B+ enzymes.
Add 19 ul of the primer kit and 5 ul of enzyme mix in solution B+.
Dispense 24 ul reaction solutions in each well.
Add 1 ul of RNA.
Spin briefly at 4°C at 3000 rpm to drop any reagents by the side of tube.
Observe the protocol for the type of run whether degenerate or non-degenerate.
Place tube with reaction mix into the Real-Time PCR machine and cycle as follows:
Reverse transcription 42°C for 45 minutes
Inactivate RT 95°C for 3 minutes
Perform PCR cycles for Degenerate primers:

    95°C for 45 seconds,
    44°C for 45 seconds,
    60°C for 45 seconds for a total of 32 cycles.

Non-degenerate primers:
(Sabin): 95°C for 45 seconds,
50°C for 45 seconds and
65°C for 45 seconds for a total of 32 cycles.

The type of fluorescein determines the type of run. Sabin multiplex uses three types of fluorescein: CY, FAM and ROX. (CY = Sabin 1, FAM = Sabin 2. and ROX =Sabin 3).

Pan Entero and Pan Polio.

Place in the qPCR machine and choose between the degenerate primer machine or the non-degenerate primer machine.

Follow the instruction on the qPCR machine to complete the run.

11. For observation and analysis of the result, follow the instruction of the set-up computer programme.

Interpretation

The Ct threshold will show from where you can then read off your result. The results are interpreted by looking for a cycle threshold value (Ct) of between 10-28. These are calculated automatically by the computer software. When the Ct value is 30, then values less than 30 are positive while values more than 30 are negative.

The polymerase chain reaction as a modern diagnostic procedure has some very good advantages. It is extremely sensitive, being able to detect down to one viral genome per sample volume. It is easy to set up and it has fast turnaround time. Many samples can be treated at relatively short time, thereby making diagnosis and therapuetic intervention fast. It also has some disadvantages. Because of the extreme sensitivity, it is liable to contamination. A very high degree of skill and proficiency is required by operators. It is often not easy to quantitate results

Further Reading

Altshuler M. *PCR Troubleshooting: The Essential guide.* Caiser Academic Press,2006 London.

John R Stephenson, Allan Warnes. *Diagnostic Virology Protocols.* Humama Press 2007.

Julie Logan, Kristin Edwards, and Nick Saunders. *Real Time PCR: Current Technology and Applications.* Caiser Academic Press, 2009, London.

McPherson M.J. And Moller S.G. PCR Springer, BIOS.

CHAPTER 9

MONOCLONAL ANTIBODIES AND THEIR PRODUCTION

One of the greatest impediments to the rapid developments of effective diagnosis of viral diseases in Nigeria is the lack of diagnostic reagents. These reagents are most of the time imported at *very high* exorbitant cost from abroad. Delays in acquiring such reagents often make diagnosis and intervention almost impossible. It is not unusual to find clinical specimens sent abroad for diagnosis for a simple test that could have been done locally were the reagents available.

One of such reagents is the monoclonal antibodies to the various prevailing viruses in the country.

Monoclonal antibodies have emerged as important diagnostic and research tools in clinical and laboratory medicine. The development of high quality monoclonal antibodies to a variety of viruses today has made the use of various serological tests more routine in many laboratories, and has contributed to the rapid detection of these viruses in clinical specimens. Specific identification of viruses can be made within hours of obtaining specimens.

Monoclonal antibody is a homogenous population of antibody molecules produced by the descendants of a single B lymphocyte. They are produced by B lymphocyte hybridomas made by fusing B lymphocytes with myeloma cells. The lymphocytes contribute specific antibody producing genes to the hybridoma while the myeloma provides genes that allow the hybridoma to divide indefinitely and continue to express the immunoglobulin genes.

The lymphocytes are obtained from animals, usually mice (Balb/C) that have been immunised with specific antigens. The Balb/C mice are usually the best breed for monoclonal antibody production because most of the myeloma cells used originate from the Balb/C mice. Most of the myeloma cells carry the murine Balb/C histocompatibility antigens. The myeloma cell line does not produce antibodies of its own. It is 8-azaguanine resistant. It is very easy to culture and is not dangerous to use; it is a mouse tumor that is not harmful to humans.

Lymphocytes and myeloma cells are fused together in medium containing polyethylene glycol and are seeded into tissue culture flasks containing peritoneal macrophages as feeder cells. The selective hypoxan thine-aminopterin-thymidine (HAT) medium allows the hybridomas to multiply into visible colonies but kills myeloma cells that have not fused with lymphocytes. The culture is tested for the presence of specific antibody. Specific antibody- producing hybridoma cultures can be expanded and cloned.

The production of monoclonal antibodies involve some specific stepwise procedures listed below:

1. Preparation of antigen for immunization

Prepare the virus stock against which the monoclonal antibody is to be prepared. This is done by growing the virus in a suitable susceptible cell line. The stock virus is titrated and quantified to determine the viral unit.

2. Immunisation of mice

(1) Record the sources and history of BALB/C mice and the myeloma cells.

(2) Immunise about 5-6 adult female mice. The purpose is to increase the number of B-lymphocytes capable of producing antibodies of desired specificity. A standard immunisation protocol is to administer a primary intraperitoneal injection of the antigen, followed by a secondary intravenous injection three weeks later.

The first injection stimulates primary antibody response and expands the number of B-lymphocytes while the second injection expands the number of specific B lymphocytes.

(3) Screen mice for specific antibody production. Use two mice with the highest antibody titre.

3. Preparation of spleen cells

(1) Aseptically remove the spleen cells in a biosafety cabinet class II into 5 ml of DMEM supplemented with 15% fetal calf serum.

(2) Chop or macerate into bits with sterile scalpels and forcepts. Pass through sterile nylon mesh to produce single spleen cell suspension.

(3) Centrifuge in a 15ml centrifuge tube at 500g for 10 minutes.

(4) Suspend pellet in 4 ml of hemolyzing solution made up of 155mM NH_4Cl, 10 mM $KHCO_3$, 1 mM Na_2EDTA, pH7.0) and keep at 0°C for 5 minutes to lyse the red blood cells.

(5) Wash off lysed RBC in 10ml of the 15% DMEM centrifuge again at 500g for 10 minutes.

(6) Wash again in plain DMEM and centrifuge as above.

(7) Count the number of spleen cells, i.e. lymphocytes.

This stage is very important for fusion with myeloma cells in the later stage.

4. Culture and preparation of myeloma cells

(1) Several myeloma cell lines are available – P3, 653, NS1 and SP2/0.

(2) A week before fusion, culture the myeloma cells in 15% DMEM supplemented with 4.5gm of glucose per liter. Add L-glutamine, antibiotics and fungizone.

(3) Incubate at 37°C in 5% CO_2. Myeloma cells can be sub-cultured every 4-5 days to keep them in log phase growth.

(4) Count the number of myeloma cells using the standard cell counting technique to determine the number of viable myeloma cells/m.

(5) To ensure 8-azaguanine resistance myeloma cells should be cultured in medium with 8-azaguanine once or twice a year.

5. Fusion of lymphocytes and Myeloma cells

(1) The fusion stage is very important. The fusion should be such that lymphocyte cells (spleen cells) are mixed with myeloma cells in the ratio of 2:1.

(2) In a conical flask/or 50ml centrifuge tube, add $1x 10^8$ spleen cells unto $5x 10^7$ of myeloma cells and add 50 ml of the HAT medium.

See Table 9.1 for the appropriate mixture of the myeloma and lymphocyte cells.

(3) Mix thoroughly in serum free prewarmed at 38°C DMEM and centrifuge again at 500g x 10 minutes.

(4) Using sterile pipette, completely aspirate supernatant and gently disrupt the pellet. Place the tube at 37°C water bath and keep it there during the fusion.

(5) Add drop wise 0.5 ml pre-warmed at 38°C 40% PEG 6000, gently and manually rotating the centrifuge tube for 1 minute to mix the PEG and cells.

(6) Add 1 ml per 30 seconds pre-warmed at 38°C DMEM without serum and rotate gently as above.

(7) Repeat 9 more times the addition of 0.5 ml pre-warmed at 40°C PEG 6000 gently while rotating the centrifuge tube for 1 minute to mix the PEG and cells.

(8) Add 20 ml 15% DMEM pre-warmed at 38°C and centrifuge at 500g for 10 minutes.

HAT medium can be prepared from a 50X HAT medium supplement using the formula:

$$C_1 V_1 = C_2 V_2$$

Where C_1 = initial concentration

$V1$ = desired volume

$C2$ = desired concentration

$V2$ = known volume

Substituting $50 X V_1$ = $1 X 50$ ml

$$V1 \quad = \quad \frac{1 \times 50 =}{50} \quad 1 \text{ ml}$$

Take 1 ml of the 50X HAT supplement, and add to 49 ml of DMEM
plus 15% Fetal Calf serum plus antibiotics.

(9) Aspirate supernatant and wash cells twice by centrifugation in
HAT medium supplemented with 15% FCS.

(10) Suspend pellet in the appropriate volume of HAT medium (see
Table 9.1).

(11) Dispense 200 ul of the hybridoma cells in flat bottom 96-well
cell culture plate.

(12) Seal and incubate at 37°C in 5% CO_2.

(13) At 2 to 3 days interval remove 100ul from each well and replace
with 100 ul HAT medium.

(14) Starting from the 8th day, exchange medium with HT medium.

(15) Monitor the growth of hybridoma. The morphologies of
hybridomas can be easily differentiated from the spleen and
myeloma cells.

(16) At about the 10th day, screen for specific MAb productivity by
ELISA or IFA.

Total No of lymphocyte	Total No of Myeloma	Amount of HAT
1×10^8	5×10^7	50 ml
9×10^7	4.5×10^7	45 ml
8×10^7	4.0×10^7	40 ml
7×10^7	3.5×10^7	35 ml
6×10^7	3.0×10^7	30 ml
5×10^7	2.5×10^7	25 ml
4×10^7	2.0×10^7	20 ml
3×10^7	1.5×10^7	15 ml

Table 9.1. Correct Mixture of Myeloma and Lymphpcyte cells

Screening for MAb producing hybridoma and cloning by limiting
Dilution

Cloning for specific MAb is done by the limiting dilution method. The
hybridomas produced initially are in a mixture of population of cells

containing non-secreting hybridomas, cells secreting antibodies of other specificities, other cells that survive HAT and antibody-secreting the desired MAbs. These cells must be separated from each other and grown in single isolated cells in culture to form a clone. Once an antibody secreting clones have been identified, they should be expanded.

Before cloning, specific MAb producing cells must be screened by ELISA.

ELISA
Procedure
(1) Prepare suspension of the antigen (e.g. Yellow Fever virus).
(2) Dispense suspension of the antigen in labelled 96-well ELISA plates.
(3) Allow to stand at room temperature for 2 hours.
(4) Wash tree times with 0.05% Tween 20-PBS.
(4) Block with a suspension of dry milk or any other blocking buffer.
(5) Add 50ul of corresponding culture supernatant of hybridoma cells to each well and allow to stand at room temperature for 1 hour.
(6) Wash three times with 0.05% Tween-PBS.
(7) Prepare a 1:200 dilution of mouse 1g-specific Ab conjugated with enzyme e.g. horse radish peroxidase.
(8) Add 50 ml of the mouse 1g to each well and allow to stand at room temperature for 1 hour.
(9) Wash three times with Tween-PBS.
(10) Add substrate to each well and allow to stand for 30 minutes at room temperature.
(11) Detect visually or by ELISA reader.
(12) Record MAb-positive well as well as MAb producing hybridomas.
(13) Mix and transfer such MAb producing hybridomas to 24 well plate for expansion.
(14) Culture in HT medium for 4-5 days.

The hybridoma cloning is performed as follows:
(1) Count the number of antibody producing hybridomas in each of the corresponding wellof the 24-well culture plate.

(2)   Place 2 x 10^4 peritoneal cells (feeder cells) of normal Balb/C mouse in each 96-well plate.

(3)   Place the plate at 37°C in 5% CO_2 while preparing the diluted suspension of hybridoma.

(4)   Prepare a suspension of hybridoma cells in HT medium to contain 100 viable cells / 10ml. This will give a final concentration of 1 cell / 0.1 ml of medium.

(5)   Dispense 0.1 ml of the hybridoma dilution into the 96 well plates. Agitate the cells frequently to keep the diluted hybridoma cells uniformly suspended in medium.

(6)   Incubate the plate at 37°C in 5% CO_2 for 4-7 days. You need not change the medium. Observe for growth of isolated clones of hybridomas cells. A true clone will be characterised by a very uniform, circular border.

(7)   The supernatants from wells containing one hybridoma clone per well can be assayed for the production of the desired antibody specificity by ELISA.

(8)   Transfer positive clones into larger volumes of medium e.g. 25 cm^2 flask.

(9)   A second cloning by limiting dilution is desirable to ensure that a true clone is produced.

(10) Freeze each MAb producing hybridoma for future recovery.

Further Reading

Albitar M. *Monoclonal Antibodies: Methods and Protocols* Humana press 1st ed. 2007.

McCollough KC, and Spier RE. *Monoclonal Antibodies in biotechnology: Theoretical and Practical Aspects*. Cambridge University Press 1st ed. 2009.

Shire SJ, Gombotz W, Bechtold –Peters, K and Andya J. *Current trends in Monoclonal Antibody Development and Manufacturing*. 1st ed. Springer 2009.

PART III

SPECIFIC VIRUS FAMILIES:
CHARACTERISTICS, IDENTIICATION
AND LABORATORY
DIAGNOSIS

RNA VIRUSES

CHAPTER 10

Family PICORNAVIRIDAE

Viruses belonging to the Picornaviridae family are the smallest of the RNA viruses, two characteristics from which the name was derived. "Pico" meaning small and "rna" denoting the type of nucleic acid. Picornaviridae consists of nine genera, namely Apthovirus, Cardiovirus, Enterovirus, Erbovirus, Hepatovirus, Kobuvirus, Parechovirus, Rhinovirus and Teschovirus. The Enteroviruses and the Rhinovirus are particularly important as agents of human diseases while the Apthovirus belongs to the Foot and Mouth Disease virus, a virus of very important veterinary significance. The Picornaviruses are all non-enveloped single stranded RNA viruses with positive polarity i.e. the viral RNA acts as the mRNA, a condition that makes the mRNA infectious.

The Enteroviruses

The Enteroviruses replicate in the alimentary tract and are therefore resistant to acidic pH, one property that differentiates them from the Rhinoviruses of the same family.

The Enteroviruses consist of about 71 serotypes made up of 3 poliovirus serotypes. Coxsackievirus A (23 serotypes), Coxsackievirus B(6 serotypes) Echovirus (28 serotypes) and Human Enterovirus (4 serotypes).

Table 10.1 Classification and properties of Enteroviruses					
Group Virus	Types	Monkey kidney	Human cell culture	Pathology in newborn mice	Major disease associations
Poliovirus	3 types (1 - 3)	+	+	-	Paralytic poliomyelitis, aseptic meningitis, febrile illness.
Coxsackie group A	23 types (A1-22, A24)	- or E	- or E	+	Aseptic meningitis, herpangina, febrile illness, conjunctivitis, hand, foot and mouth disease.
Coxsackie group B	6 types (B1-6)	+	+	+	Aseptic meningitis, severe neonatal disease, myopericarditis, Bornholm disease, encephalitis, febrile illness
Echovirus	31 types (1-9, 11-27)	+	E	-	Aseptic meningitis, rash, febrile illness, conjunctivitis, severe generalized neonatal disease.
+ *Positive, - Negative, E CPE non visible(Eclipse)*					

Table 10.1 Classification and properties of Enteroviruses

Although they inhabit alimentary tract, their target organs are not limited to the gastrointestinal tract alone, but often involve the central nervous system. They cause a variety of clinical syndromes ranging from poliomyelitis (poliovirus) to aseptic meningitis, myorcarditis and pericarditis.

Entrovriruses are all similar in their structures. They are between 25-30 nm in diameter with icosahedral symmetry and possess 32 capsomeres and about 60 protomeres each of which contains the nonglycosylated virus proteins VP1, VP2, VP3 and VP4. VP1, VP2 and VP3 are located exterior to the capsid while the VP4 is located in the interior of the capsid. These virus proteins play a major role in the molecular characteristic and identification of the different genotypes and serotypes.

Host Range

Human is the natural host of the poliovirus although primate monkeys can be successfully infected. Antibody to polio virus has been found in monkeys and other non-human primates. The poliovirus can be readily isolated in tissue culture cells. Hep2C, Rhabdyomyosarcoma cells (RD) are the most commonly used cells until recently when the L20B cell, a genetically engineered cell line to which the polio receptor CD-155 has been incorporated, was developed. One good advantage of the L20B cell is its specificity to poliovirus. Only poliovirus (except some few Adenoviruses) will grow in L20B cell lines, while polio and other enteroviruses will grow in Hep-2C and RD.

Coxsackievirus will grow in new born mice. Group A and B coxsackie viruses can be distinguished by the distinct pathology they cause in mice.

Sources of specimen and specimen collection

Stool is the best specimen for the isolation of enterovirus in cell culture, although the virus can be found in the blood and cerebrospiral fluid. Stool is the specimen of choice for the following reasons: the virus is found in its highest titre in the stool, the consistency of the stool protects the virus from desiccation and stool can easily be obtained without having to resort to invasive procedure. Because of the shedding pattern of the virus, two stool samples taken at 24 hours interval should be taken.

In the absence of stool, rectal swabs and throat swab can be considered. Specimens for virus isolation should be transported to the lab in reverse cold chain.

Stool Preparation for virus isolation

The procedure of processing the stool removes the organic materials, bacteria, fungi, parasites and other enveloped viruses from the specimen. This is achieved through chloroform treatment:

Procedure

1. Add 2-3 g of stool into the 50 ml centrifuge tube.
2. Add 10 ml of cold PBS.
3. Add 5 ml of laboratory grade chloroform.
4. Add enough of glass beads.
5. Screw cap and shake vigorously manually or mechanically with the glass beads for 20 minutes in a mechanical shaker.
6. Spin at 3000 rpm for 10 minutes in a cold centrifuge (4-8°C).
7. With a sterile pipette, aspirate the aqueous layer containing the virus and dispense 0.2 ml in 2.5 ml cryovial. Store away at -20°C until ready for inoculation (See Fig. 4.2).

Virus inoculation and propagation in cell culture

Before stool preparation, monolayer of RD, Hep2-C, and L20B cell lines must have been grown in tissue culture tubes or 25 cm² tissue culture flasks.

Procedure

1. Gently pour off the growth medium from the cell monolayer.
2. Inoculate between 0.1 – 0.2 ml of virus suspension.
3. Incubate at 37oC for 1 hour.
4. Add about 2 ml of maintenance medium and incubate at 37oC.
5. Check for evidence of viral growth daily. Cytopathic effect will usually be observed in inoculated cells in 24 – 70 hours if the stool contains the virus. Enterovirus cytopathic effect is characterised by cell rounding.
6. Instead of stage 1 above, the virus can be inoculated directly into the just seeded cells in growth medium. This is referred to as the 'wet inoculation'.

Although most coxsackie viruses will grow in cell cultures, isolation from clinical specimen may not be successful always. As stated above, virus isolation can be achieved in new born suckling mice.

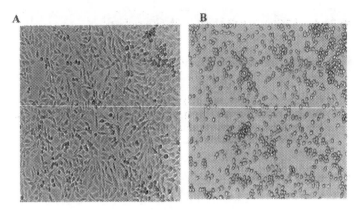

Fig 10.1 L20B Cell. **(A)**Uninfected **(B)** Infected with poliovirus showin 4+CPE

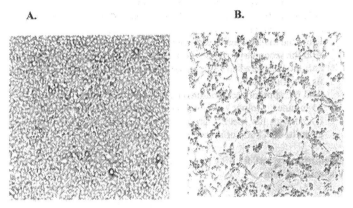

Fig.10.2. RD cells. (A) Uninfected (B) infected with enterovirus showing 3+CPE

Entero Virus Identification and Typing

The existence of many serotypes of enteroviruses used to pose some problems with identification of the various serotypes. However, the current global polio eradication initiative (PEI) has drawn attention to and has facilitated the laboratory diagnosis of these viruses through a network of global laboratories. Enteroviruses can now be easily identified using the standard neutralization test according to the WHO recommended protocol (WHO Manual for the virologic investigation of poliomyelitis WHO/EPI/GEN/02.1.2002, Geneva, Switzerland) and also by the molecular serotyping technique as described by the CDC, (Oberste et al. 2003).

Poliovirus can be differentiated from other enteroviruses through its selective growth in L20B. However a confirmation test will be required for final identification. Also, a presumptive diagnosis of other enteroviruses can be made based on their susceptibility differences in different cell lines.

The Global Polio Laboratory Network

The Global Polio Eradication Initiative (PEI) is supported by a well knit Global Polio Laboratory Network (GPLN) which is organised into three levels based on their activities and responsibilities. These are the National Laboratories (NL), the Regional Reference Laboratories (RRL) and the Global Specialized Laboratories.

The National Laboratories accept and process stools, undertake the initial virus inoculation, isolation, identification and typing into serotypes. The NL refers the poliovirus isolates to the Regional Reference laboratories and at the same time reports isolation and serotype results to the programme and field investigators.

The Regional Reference Laboratories (RRL) The RRLs perform intratypic differentiation test on isolates referred from the NLs. The intratypic test differentiates between the wild circulating poliovirus and the vaccine (Sabin) strains. Two types of tests – an antigenic, the Enzyme linked immunosorbent assay (ELISA) and a molecular (RT-PCR or Probe Hybridization test), are used for intratypic differentiation. The RRLs also distribute reference materials such as antisera and cell lines to the NLs. One major responsibility of the RRL is to immediately report the intratypic test result to the field investigators and the immunisation group while at the same time referring the wild and Sabin viruses to the Specialized Laboratories for sequencing.

The Global Specialized Laboratories (GSLs) The main function of the GSL is to give a final definitive identification of the poliovirus using all available techniques including genetic characterisation, and sequencing. Results of tests performed at the GSL allow for ability to detect origin of isolates, path of transmission of isolates, reservoirs and circulation patterns and the general epidemiology of the virus. These are particularly important because this information guides the programme as well as determine the success and failure of the immunisation and surveillance. The GSLs prepare and distribute proficiency panels for the assessment of activities of the NL and RRL and also take part in the training of technical staff of the Network. The Global Polio Laboratory Network (GPLN) has formed the basis for laboratory investigation and coordination of other future eradication programme and integrated disease surveillance (IDS). The experience gained through the GPLN should form a very strong link between laboratory and disease surveillance in terms of specimen transportation, specimen processing, characterisation of infectious agents, regular reporting of results and maintenance of high laboratory performance standard.

Cell lines for isolation and identification of poliovirus and other enteroviruses

Poliovirus will grow in a variety of cell lines such as Vero, Hep-2C, RD and L20B. However, two cell lines – the RD and L20B have been specifically selected by the WHO for the purpose of isolation and identification.

L20B

The L20B cell line is a genetically engineered murine cell line to which the poliovirus receptor CD155 gene has been transfected. The unique advantage of this cell line is that it only supports the growth of poliovirus which produces the type specific enterovirus CPE characterised by cell rounding. Some adenoviruses and reoviruses may cause CPE in L20B. The type of grapelike CPE produced is however easily distinguished from the rounding nature seen with the enteroiruses.

A small number of non-polio enteroviruses e.g. Coxsackie A virus may also show CPE in this cell line. This is rare and is usually not noticed in primary isolation but after previous isolation of such coxsackie A virus in another cell line.

RD

The rhabdomyosarcoma cell line (RD) is derived from the human rhabdomyosarcoma. This cell line supports the growth of both poliovirus and other enteroviruses producing the characteristic enterovirus CPE.

The use of L20B and RD provides great sensitivity and specificity in the isolation of poliovirus.

Isolation of poliovirus and other enteroviruses
Material
Tissue culture tubes of confluent L20B and RD cell lines.
2% MEM.
1, 5ml disposable pipettes.
Procedure
Seed a known concentration of both cell lines into two tissue culture tubes
Examine the two cell lines for confluency and healthy growth. Cells are best inoculated 48 hours after seeding.
Decant the growth medium and replace with 1ml maintenance medium.
Label two tubes for L20B and RD for each specimen (see stool extraction) indicating specimen number, date of inoculation and passage number.
Provide one tube each for cell control.
Inoculate 0.2ml of the specimen and incubate tubes in stationary slanting position at 36°C.
Examine culture daily for CPE with the inverted microscope for CPE.
Record CPE or no CPE in all inoculated and control tubes for 7 days.
Depending on the degree of CPE. mark +1 - +4 indicating from 25% CPE to 100% CPE.
Store all those tubes showing up to 3+ or 75% CPE at -20°C.
Do second passage by passing the isolate into another L20B or RD depending on which cell line the virus was originally isolated.

In the absence of CPE in the first passage, perform a blind passage by inoculating into another tube of confluent cell and examine for another 7 days.

Inoculate RD positive but L20B negative cells into L20B cells and examine for 7 days.

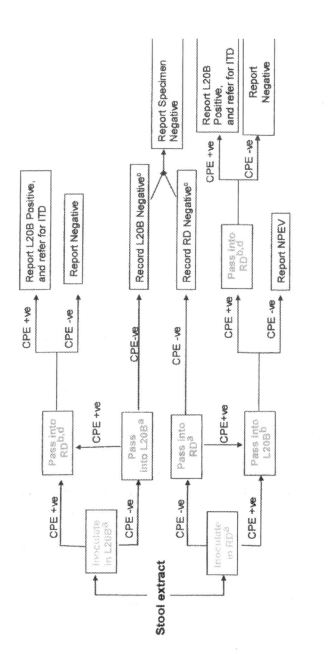

Fig – 10.3 Flow Chart for Poliovirus isolation in RD and L20B cells *(Adapted from the WHO Polio Manual, 4ᵗʰ ed. WHO Geneva, 2004 S1. Supplement to the WHO Polio Manual with permission)*

a   observed for a minimum of 5 days.
b   until 3+ CPE obtained (usually 1-2 days, 5 days maximum)
c   Total minimum observation time of 10 days
d   Pool L20B positive tubes (if more than one) before final RD passage

Identification and serotyping of Poliovirus Isolates

The different serotypes of polioviruses are identified from the isolated polioviruses using the micro neutralisation test. Polyclonal antisera against the types 1, 2, and 3 polioviruses are used in this neutralisation test. These antisera are supplied by the National Institute of Public Health and Environment (RIVM), Beethoven, The Netherlands. The poliovirus microneutralisation test is the Beta method which utilises constant virus dilution of 10^3 and 10^4 against 1:128 of the various polio pool monospecific polyclonal antisera (polio 1,2,3, polio 1,2 polio 1,3 and polio 2,3). This mixture of virus/antibody is incubated for 1 hour at 36°C to allow the antibodies to bind to the virus. Cell suspensions are then added to the well plates and examined daily for presence or absence of CPE. The antiserum pools that prevent the development of CPE indicate the identity of the virus isolate or mixtures of the viruses. The non-replication of a virus in the presence of a pool of antisera is because the infectivity of the virus was neutralised by one of the antisera component present in the pool.

For further information on the identification and serotyping of poliovirus by neutralisation test, the interested reader is referred to the WHO Polio Manual (WHO Manual for the virologic investigation of poliomyelitis WHO/EPI/GEN/02.1.2002, Geneva, Switzerland).

Intratypic Differentiation of Polioviruses

Epidemiologically, three types of the poliovirus circulate. These are: The vaccine strain, usually referred to as the Sabin like (SL). The SL circulates widely during and after immunisation campaigns and can be found in healthy and symptomatic children.

The wild strain referred to as Non-Sabin-like (NSL) is mostly responsible for the AFP cases.

The circulating vaccine-derived poliovirus (cVDPV) which is a revertant. The cVDPVs are often found in areas of low vaccine coverage and where the previous wild type has been eradicated. The cVDPV has lost the attenuation of the OPV strain and has therefore acquired neurovirulence observed with the NSL strain, as a result of a change in the neucleotide from A to G in position 481 of the 5/ UTR region.

It is therefore necessary to determine whether a given poliovirus isolate is one of these three.

Five intratypic methods are currently in use for this differentiation; however the GPLN supports three, one antigenic method which is the ELISA and one molecular, which could either be the Probe Hybridization test or the Polymerase Chain Reaction (PCR).

ELISA

The ELISA test for intratypic differentiation is performed only on single serotype isolates. Mixtures should therefore be first separated into their respective serotypes by growing the isolate in the presence of the appropriate antisera.

The ELISA technique for the intratypic differentiation of poliotypes pathoypes and serotypes has been excellently described in the WHO Polio Laboratory manual 4th Edition 2004(WHO 2004). Interested reader is advised to consult this book.

Polymerase Chain Reaction(PCR) for Intratypic differentiation of poliovirus

The PCR is one of the molecular methods for intratypic differentiation of poliovirus. The test is done on the virus after it has been identified. The viral RNA is converted into complementary DNA (cDNA) by reverse transcriptase. The PCR products are resolved by gel electrophoresis. Three sets of specific primers are used. These include primers for enterovirus group, primers for Sabin type specific group for each of the 3 serotypes, primers for all poliovirus group and all isolates of the 3 serotypes. This set of primers will identify all poliovirus isolates and confirm the serotypes. The PCR kits are supplied by the Centers for Disease Control and Prevention and consist of the followings:

1. Box *One*
(a) Four vials of primers in Buffer A (serotype 1, 2, 3, Sabins).

(b) Positive controls for each primer set (four vials).

(c) Multiplex Sabin-specific primers combined in a single reaction.

2. Box *Two*

(a) Two vials of primers in Buffer A (Pan-entero and Pan Polio).

(b) Control for each primer set (two vials).

3. Box *Three*

(a) Six vials of Buffer B.

DTT and enzyme should be added prior to use.

(b) One vial of DTT.

(c) One vial of 1X PCR buffer for diluting DNA molecular marker.

(d) One copy of package insert.

The enzymes, RNase, AMV reverse transcriptase (RT) and Taq Polymerase are supplied separately. Other reagents needed include the molecular marker, 6X gel loading dye, ethidium bromide (1mg/ml) and nuclease free water.

Like the ELISA method for intratypic differentiation of poliovirus, the PCR method has been well described in the WHO polio manual (WHO,2002, 2004) from where additional information on the procedures, reagents, interpretation of results etc, can be obtained.

ITD Probe Hybridisation Method

The Probe Hybridisation Test is the second molecular method recommended by WHO for intratypic differentiation between the wild and sabin polioviruses.

The poliovirus RNA is extracted and immobilised onto filters. Digoxygenin – labelled enterovirus group, sabin type-specific and wild virus genotype-specific probes are added and allowed to hybridise to the immobilised RNA. After washing to remove unbound probes, the bound probe is then detected by using a colorimetric reagent.

Probe Hybridisation Kit consists of the followings reagents that are also developed and supplied by the Centers for Disease Control and Prevention, Atlanta, Georgia, USA.

Digoxygenin (DIG) labelled RNA probe consisting of Enterovirus group, Sabin 1, Sabin 2, Sabin 3.

Unlabelled non-infectious positive control RNA transcripts containing the three Sabin strain sequences (Sabin 1, Sabin 2 and Sabin 3).

Three wild poliovirus negative control RNAs (W1, W2, W3).

The RNA probes are resuspended in 20μl of nuclease-free distilled water.

For further understanding of the procedure, interpretation of results readers are advised to consult the WHO Polio Manual (WHO 2002, 2004).

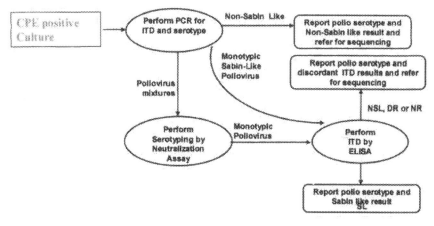

- CPE positive cultures represent 2 categories of isolates: L20B+RD+ or RD+L20B+RD+
- L20B+RD+ isolates are always tested by PCR
- RD+L20B+RD+are only tested in limited situations
  - if this is the only isolate obtained from the specimen
  - if the corresponding L20B+RD+ isolate gives a non-polio or non-entero PCR result

Fig.10. 4 Flow chart for the intratypic differentiation of poliovirus
(Reproduced with permission from the S1. Supplement to the WHO Polio Manual,4th *ed. WHO Geneva, 2004*

Festus D. Adu

Circulating Vaccine Derived polioviruses(cVDPV) and their Laboratory Identification

Vaccine derived polioviruses (VDPV) are poliovirus isolates having >1% nucleotide sequence divergence from the Sabin strain in the ~900 nucleotide (nt) region encoding the major capsid proteins VP1 (Kew et al 2005, CDC 2002). It is a rare strain of poliovirus that has genetically mutated from the strain contained in the oral polio vaccine (OPV), the weakened or attenuated version of the poliovirus used for the immunisation against the wild poliovirus outbreak. When this rare strain of the poliovirus acquire the ability of circulating and spreading within the population and causing paralytic poliomyelitis, it is referred to as circulating vaccine derived poliovirus (cVDPV) to differentiate it from other VDPVs. The extensive use of the OPV has succeeded in reducing the incidences of paralytic poliomyelitis caused by the wild poliovirus worldwide. However, replication of the OPV in the human gut can be accompanied by some genetic changes of the vaccine virus. These changes may include reversion of the attenuating mutations and intratypic and intertypic recombinations with other enteroviruses or OPV strains. The emergence of cVDPV is often enhanced by (1) low vaccination coverage which often results in low level population immunity. Nearly all cVDPVs occur in an environment of poor OPV coverage and where gaps in population immunity have been established for one reason or the other and the corresponding wild poliovirus strain has been eradicated. (2) Poor sanitation which may include wide population density, poor hygiene and overcrowding and (3) tropical conditions.

Circulating vaccine derived polioviruses share some similarities with the wild polioviruses.

Like the wild polioviruses, cVDPVs have the capacity for sustained person to person transmission.

cVDPVs have a significant attack rates close to those of the wild polioviruses

They are highly neurovirulent for transgenic mice.

They replicate at supraoptimal temperature of 39.5^0C.

They undergo recombination with other non-polio entero-viruses

Laboratory Identification of cVDPVs

Poliovirus isolates for VDPV screening

All suspected poliovirus isolate cultures which had earlier been tested and found to be Sabin –like must be screened for cVDPV. Monotypic Sabin-like poliovirus isolates must be screened for VDPV while poliovirus mixtures must be first separated into their monotypes by neutralisation. However the use of real time PCR has made mixture seperation unnecessary.

cVDPV Identification

ELISA

The initial identification of cVDPV was by the ELISA test, where the result of the test may flag the virus as double reactive (DR), non reactive (NR) or invalid. However, the ELISA test now seems inadequate because a very high percentage of cVDPVs are not flagged as cVDPV even after many nucleotide changes from the original Sabin virus. (Table 10.2). Therefore the ELISA test is fast being replaced by the qPCR. Table 10.2 shows the result of ELISA tests performed on 10 Nigerian poliovirus isolates. Result of ITD ELISA showed that eight of the ten suspected polio isolates were type-2 Sabin-like polioviruses while two had invalid results. VDPV VP1 and 3D polassays however flagged all the isolates as Non-Sabin- like. All the ten isolates turned out to be type -2 cVDPVs after sequencing.

ELISA ASSAY

EPID No.	Isolation Result	ITD ELISA	cVDPV qPCR	3D Pol PCR
NIE-NIS-KNT-09-001	SP	SL-2	NSL	NSL
NIE-ZAS-BKA-09-002	SP	SL-2	NSL	NSL
NIE-ZAS-ANK-09-003	SP	SL-2	NSL	NSL
NIE-KBS-DKG-O8-007	SP	SL-2	NSL	NSL
NIE-KDS-GKW-09-001	SP	SL-2	NSL	NSL
NIE-ZAS-SKF-08-014	SP	INVALID	NSL	NSL
NIE-NIS-RJA-09-001	SP	SL-2	NSL	NSL
NIE-ZAS-BKA-09-003	SP	SL-2	NSL	NSL
NIE-ZAS-GMM-08-015	SP	SL-2	NSL	NSL
NIE-ZAS-GMM-08-016	SP	INVALID	NSL	NSL

EPID   =   Epidemiological number
SP   =   Suspected polio
ITD ELISA   =   Intratypic differentiation Enzyme linked
                            Immunosorbent assay
cVDPV   =   circulating vaccine derived poliovirus
qPCR   =   quantitative polymerase chain reaction
SL   =   Sabin-like
NSL   =   Non Sabin-like

Table 10.2 Showing the discrepancies between ELISA test and the Real Time PCR in the identification of cVDPV.

Real time PCR
The Centres for Disease Control and Prevention, Atlanta Georgia, USA has developed a highly sensitive and specific primers and assays

for the accurate screening and identification of cVDPVs. These primers are directed against the VP1 and the 3D pol regions of the virus. (Details of the tests have been described briefly in the earlier chapter of this book. The interested reader who needs more details is advised to read further any of the selected literature cited at the end of this chapter).

A positive cVDPV result will give a negative amplification result both with the VP1 assay and the 3D pol VDPV assay or a negative VP1 VDPV assay and a positive 3D pol VDPV assay. A positive amplification in both the VP1 and 3D pol assay confirms a Sabin-like isolate (Table 10.3).

Sequencing
Isolates suspected to be VDPVs must be referred for sequencing. The sequence analysis will determine the number of nucleotide changes and degree of divergence from the original Sabin virus.
Depending on the period the virus has been in circulation, the number of nucleotide changes may vary from as low as 5 to as high as 40 nucleotide changes from the original Sabin virus.

VP1	3D	Result	Comments
+	+	SL	Report SL
+	-	SL	Report SL
-	+	NSL	Report NSL and refer for sequencing
-	-	NSL	Report NSL and refer for sequencing

+ = Amplification
− = No amplification
SL = Sabin-like
NSL = Non-Sabin-like

Table 10.3. Interpretation VDPV assay results

Further Reading
Adu, F.D., Iber Jane, Bukbuk D., Harry, T., Gumede, N., Yang, S-J et al. 2007. "Isolation of Recombinant Type-2 Vaccine Derived Poliovirus from a Nigerian child." *Virus Res 127:17-25.*

Chen –Fu Yang, Tary Naguib, Su-Ju Yang, Eman Nasr, Jaume Jorba et al. 2003. "Circulation of Endemic Type -2 Vaccine Derived Poliovirus in Egypt from 1983-1993."*J. Virol 77 (15) : 8366 - 8377*

David R. Kilpatrick, Chen-Fu Yang, Karen Ching, Annelet Vincent, Jane Iber et al. "Rapid Group- Serotype- and Vaccine Strtain-specific Identification of Poliovirus Isolates by Real-time Reverse Transcription-PCR Using Degenerate Primers And Probes Containing Deoxyinosine Residues. *J. Clin Microbiol 2009*; vol 47 No 6: 1939-1941.

Hiroyuki Shimizu, Bruce Thorley, Fem Julia Paladin, Keri Anne Brussen et al. 2004. "Circulation of Type-1Vaccine Derived Polikovirus in the Philippines in 2001." *J. of Virology:*Vol 78 No24:13512-13521.

Kilpatrick, D.R., B. Nottay, C-F Yang, S-J Yang, M.N. Mulders et al. "Group-specific Identification of Polioviruses by PCR Using Primers Containing Mixed-Based or Deoxyinosine Residues in Position of Codon Degeneracy. 1996. *J. Clin Microbiol.34: 2990-2996.*

Kilpatrick, D.R., B. Nottay, C-F. Yang, S-J Yang et al. "Serotype Specific Identification of Polioviruses by PCR Using Primers Containing Mixed Based of Deoxyinosine Residues at Positions of Codon Degeneracy. *J. Clin Microbiol 1998 36:352-357.*

Kilpatrick, D.R., K. Ching, J. Iber, R. Campagnoli et al. "Multiplex PCR Method for Identifying recombinant vaccine related polioviruses. 2004" *J. Clin Microbiol. 42; 4313-4315*

Olen Kew, Victoria Morris-Glasgow, Mauricia Landerverde, Cara Burns et al. "Outbreak of Poliomyelitis in Hispaniola Associated with Circulating Type 1 Vaccine-derived poliovirus. 2002. *Science; vol 296:355-359.*

U.S. Department of Health and Human Services. Intratypic Differentiation of polioviruses by Real-time RT-PCR: Ibadan Real-Time Poliovirus ITD Training, 2009. US Department of Health and Human Resources, Public Health Services, Centers for Disease Control and Prevention.

World Health Organization. *Polio Laboratory Manual* 4th ed. "Immunization Vaccines and Biological." WHO Geneva, Switzerland, 2004.

Identification of non-polio enteroviruses using antibody neutralisation test

The large number of serotypes of non-polio enteroviruss makes it impossible to individually perform neutralisation tests on each serotype. Antisera have therefore been pooled together which allows many viruses to be identified in as far as nine tests.

Enterovirus isolates can be confirmed as specific enterovirus by neutralisation with these type specific antisera. There are at least 66 different known non-polio enteroviruses. Using individual reference antisera for individual identification is impracticable. Therefore, type specific antisera are combined in intersecting pools in such a way that antibody to one type is present in limited number of pools. The results are interpreted with a list of neutralisation patterns (Table 10.4). The pooled antisera are prepared in horse at the National Institute of Public Health and Environment (RIVM), Bithoven, The Netherlands and can be obtained through the WHO. Each box of the RIVM enterovirus typing antisera contains anti-enterovirus pools A, B, C, D, E, F and G, an anti coxsackie B virus pool and a trivalent antipolio virus pool. Before use, the antiserum pools should be diluted 1:20.

Neutralization antisera/Pattern	Virus serotype
AB	ECHO 4
AC	ECHO 7
AD	ECHO 11
AE	ECHO 14
AF	ECHO 9
AG	ECHO 6
BC	Cox A 9
BD	ECHO 1
BE	ECHO 27
BF	ECHO 3
BG	ECHO 25
CD	ECHO 21
CE	ECHO 22
CF	ECHO 2
CG	ECHO 5
DE	ECHO 20
DF	ECHO 12
DG	ECHO 30
EF	ECHO 33
EG	ECHO 29
FG	ECHO 13

Table 10.4 Enterovirus neutralisation pattern for serotyping

For further information on the identification and serotyping of the non- poliovirus enteroviruses by neutralisation test, the interested reader is refered to the WHO Polio Manual (WHO Manual for the virologic investigation of poliomyelitis WHO/EPI/GEN/02.1.2002,a Geneva, Switzerland).

Procedure for non-polio enterovirus microneutralisation test
This test is performed in a 96-well tissue culture plate according to the WHO protocol (WHO, 2002). Each unknown virus must be tested in duplicate against a trivalent pooled polio antiserum (PP), a coxsackie A9 and 20 echoviruses (A-G).

Procedure
Label the edge of the microtitre plate as appropriate.
Add 50ul of antisera to the appropriate wells in 1-9.

Add 50ul medium to virus control wells in columns 10 rows A-D.
Prepare I0^{-2} dilution of virus.

Add 50ul virus to all wells in column 1-10 of rows A-B of sample 1
and rows C and D for sample 2.

Perform back titration of virus 1 in rows E and F and virus 2 in rows
G and H.

Cover plate and incubate for 1 hour at 36°C.

Add 100ul of RD cell lines diluted to contain 1.5 x 10^{-5} cells per
ml.

Incubate at 36°C in an atmosphere of 5% CO_2 or alternatively, seal
with a non-toxic sealer.

Examine daily for CPE until 24 hours after CPE in virus control
wells have reached 100%.

Viruses are identified following the inhibition patterns by the
antiserum pools (Table 10.4).

Molecular Techniques

The molecular methods for enterovirus identification detects
enterovirus in clinical specimens. Three categories of molecular
methods are applicable to enterovirus identification: The PCR which
is used to detect enterovirus in clinical specimen, cell culture or
biopsy; the probe hybridisation for detection and characterisation and
the genomic sequencing for specific characterisation of the viruses.

The basis for virus identification by the molecular method is the
knowledge of the sequence of the particular viral genome, because all
the determinants for their biological properties are encoded within
the nucleic acid sequence. Information provided by the nucleic acid
sequence of a virus represents its characterisation. It is now possible
to use the sequence information to assign an enterovirus isolate to a
particular serotype because the antigenic properties of these viruses
that identify them as serotypes are actually the properties of the viral
capsid proteins. This method, called molecular typing, is based on
RT-PCR and nucleotide sequencing of the 3$^{/}$ region of the entire
VP1 region.

Result of molecular serotyping by the RT-PCR can be interpreted as follows:

VP1 nucleotide identity $\geq$ 70% (>85%) = serotype
VP1 nuclerotide identity <70% = an unknown new serotype
VPI nucleotide identity between 70% and 75% = indeterminate and requires further characterisation.

Molecular Serotyping of Enteroviruses.
The neutralisation test for the typing of enteroviruses has some limitations, the chief of which is the inability of the available overlapping antisera to identify all the 66 serotypes. Only 40 can be successfully identified by this method leading to many "untypeables". Apart from this, the genetic diversity of enterovirus isolates makes their neutralisation by antiserum to the homologous prototype strain almost impossible. The molecular serotyping technique developed by Oberste and Nix of the Respiratory and Enterovirus unit of the Centers for Disease Control in Atlanta was used to overcome these limitations. The method uses five sets of primers to successfully amplify all the known 66 serotypes as well as the putative new enterovirus serotypes (Oberste et al, 2003, Nix et al 2006). Because of the genetic similarities among the enterovirus serotypes molecular methods such as the polymerase chain reaction, PCR, can be used for the detection and serotype identification. Primers constructed from the conserved sequences are used in RT-PCR assays to identify almost all the enteroviruses including the untypeable isolates. (Hyypia et al 1997).
The serotype of the enterovirus is determined by the neutralizing epitopes located in the surface of the virus capsid protein, especially the VP1 but also the VP2 and VP3(Minor et al. 1986). The VP1 gene encoding the structural protein is therefore preferred as the region for amplification by PCR, and is used as surrogate for antigenic typing (Oberste et al. 1999 a, b; d). This VP1 codes for the major antigenic sites and the most important serotype specific neutralization epitopes.

A brief description of the procedure is given below:
    1. Extract viral RNA from the virus isolate.

2. Perform in-vitro amplification of viral RNA sequence by RT-PCR or seminested RT – PCR.
3. Run the gel electrophoresis of your PCR product.
4. Visualise the PCR product in the gel under the translumincent UV lamp.
5. Cut the desired bands and purify the PCR products.
6. Run the sequence reaction of the PCR product.
7. Purify the sequence product using the Centri-SEP kit column hydration.
8. Perform the sequencing using the sequence machine AB1 3100 Genetic Analyser (Applied Biosynthesis).
9. Cleanse the sequences by trimming, and correcting the ambiguities.
10. Do the serotype analysis and determine the identity of the serotypes using the available computer programme. A partial VP-1 sequence identify score of at least 75% to any enterovirus prototype strain indicates that the isolate is of the homologous serotype, if the second highest identity score is less than 70% (Oberste et al 1999a, b. 2003).
11. Construct a phylogenetic tree to observe relationship between other enteroviruses.

Further Reading

Maher, K Kilpatrick D.R. and Pallansch M. A. 1999b "Molecular evolution of Human Enteroviruses Correlation of Serotype with VP1 Sequence and Application to Picornavirus Classification." *Journal of Virology 73:1941-1948.*

Nix W.A Oberste M.S. and Pallansch M.A. 2006. "Sensitive, Seminested PCRamplification of VP1sequence for Direct Identification of all Enterovirus Serotypes from Original Clinical Specimens." *Journal of clinical Microbiology 44(8)001-007.*

Oberste M.S. Maher K., Kilpatrick D.R. et al. 1999a. Typing of Human Enteroviruses by Partial Sequencing of VP1. *Journal of Clinical Microbiology 37: 1288-1293.*

Penranda S. Maher, K et al. "Complete Genome Sequences of all Members of the Species Human Enterovirus A." *Journal of General Virology 85.*

World Health Organization. *Manual for the Virologic Investigation of Poliomyelitis* WHO/EPI/GEN/02.1.2002 Geneva, Switzerland).

World Health Organization. *Polio Laboratory Manual 4*[th]*ed. Immunization Vaccines and Biological. WHO Geneva, Switzerland. 2004.*

World Health Organization. *Supplement to the WHO Polio Manual,* 4th *ed. WHO Geneva, 2004*

THE RHINOVIRUSES

The Rhinoviruses are the major causes of upper respiratory illness (common cold). There are 103 serotypes of Rhinoviruses made up of 100 human and 3 bovine serotypes. Instability of the rhinoviruses to lower acidic pH differentiates them from the other members of the Picornaviridae family.

The rhinoviruses are more species-specific and are more fastidious to grow in cell culture. Efficient growth occurs only on cells of human and primate origin and at optimum temperature of 33°C with rotation. Many human cells are available but by far the most commonly used are the WI-38, MRC-5, a diploid fibroblast, fetal tonsil and some strains of the HeLa cells, but the best isolation result can be achieved when various cells are inoculated at the same time. Growth in cell monolayer is characterised by rounding and aggregation similar to the enterovirus CPE.

A   B

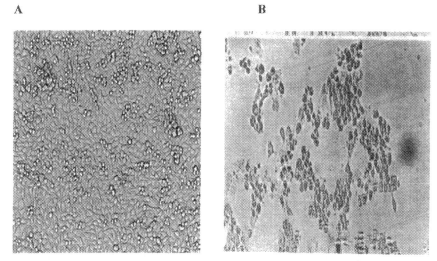

Fig.10.5 HeLa Cell. (A)uninfected (B) infected with Rhinovirus

Specimen Source and Collection

Rhinoviruses can be isolated from nasopharyngeal lavage or swabs. Specimen must be collected and inoculated immediately without freezing into cell culture for best result. In which case cells must be made available immediately after specimen collection. Inoculated cells must be rotated in roller drums to achieve maximum success.

Virus Isolation and Identification

Inoculated cells must be observed daily for evidence of virus specific CPE, which can be detected the second or third day after inoculation. Cultures should, however, be observed for about 14 days in the absence of early CPE.

The first attempt at identifying the virus is by test of liability at pH of 3. Rhinovirus, when treated at pH 3 will decrease by 2-4 logs in titre when compared with the untreated virus. However the isolate must also be tested for ether sensitivity to rule out other viruses that are also pH sensitive. The Acid-pH stability test is done as shown:

Acid –pH Stability Test
Procedure
Dilute 5ml of 0.2M tris buffer solution (pH7.4) with conc. HCl to obtain pH 3. Make up solution to 20 mls with distilled water.
Make a 1:10 dilution of the isolate with the pH 3 buffer.
Make another 1:10 dilution of virus in a pH 7 buffer.
Keep both mixtures at room temperature for 3 hours.
Make a 10 fold dilutions of both mixtures and inoculate separately 6 well per dilution.
Calculate the infectivity titres of both mixtures by the method of Reed and Muench.
A decrease in titre of 2-4 logs in the mixture treated with pH 3 buffer compared to the mixture treated with pH 7 buffer is indicative of low acid pH sensitivity. The low pH sensitive virus must however be tested for ether sensitivity to rule out other sensitive viruses that are also pH sensitive.

PCR Identification of Rhinovirus
The development of specific primers for the identification of rhinoviruses is a good alternative between enteroviruses and rhinoviruses. PCR can now detect directly rhinovirus RNA in clinical samples.

Serological Test
The existence of many serotypes of rhinoviruses has not made serological tests popular in the laboratory diagnosis of rhinoviruses. Unlike the enteroviruses, there are very few cross-reacting antigens between the serotypes. Notwithstanding, neutralisation test in culture tubes or plaque reduction neutralisation test have been used to identify some strains of the virus and for detecting serological response.
A sensitive rhinovirus antibody capture antigen ELISA can detect viral IgG and IgA in the serum.

Further reading

1. Arruda E, Pitkaranta A, Witek TJ Jr., et al. "Frequency and Natural History of Rhinovirus Infections in Adults during Autumn. *J Clin Microbiol 1997; 35: 2864-2868.*

2. Atmar RL, Guy E, Auntupalli KK, et al. "Respiratory Tract Viral Infections in Innercity Asthmatic Adults." *Arch intern Med 1998; 158; 2453-2459.*

3. Barclay WS, Al Nakib W. "An ELISA for the Detection of Rhinovirus Specific Antibody in Semen and Nasal Secretion." J Virol Methods 1987; 53-64.

4. Hyypia T, Puhakka T, Ruuskanen O, et al. "Molecular Diagnosis of Human Rhinovirus Infections: Comparison with Virus Isolation." *J Clin Microbiol 1998; 36: 2081-2083.*

5. Johnston SL, Sanderson G, Pattemore PK, et al. "Use of Polymerase Chain Reaction for Diagnosis of Prcornavirus Infection in Subjects with and without Respiratory Symptoms." *Clin Microbiol 1993; 1: 111-117.*

6. Nicholson KG, KentJ, Hammersley V, et al. "Acute Viral Infections of Upper Respiratory Tract in Elderly People Living in the Community: Comparative, Prospective, Population Based Study of Disease Burden." Br Med J 1997; 315: 1060 – 1064.

CHAPTER 11

Family PARAMYXOVIRIDAE

To the Paramyxoviridae family belong some viruses of both human and veterinary importance. Measles, mump, parainfluenza and respiratory syncytia viruses and a recently identified human virus, Nipah virus are all very important viral agents of human diseases while rinderpest of large ungulates, pestes des petit ruminants (PRR) of small ruminant and the New Castle disease virus of poultry all belong to the family paramyxoviridae. Paramyxoviridae is further divided into 2 subfamilies- the paramyxovirinae and the Pneumovirinae. The paramyxoviruses are non-segmented single stranded negative polarity enveloped RNA viruses, closely associated in their biological properties with the Orthomyxoviridae viruses in their possession of H and N genes. The presence or absence of the glycoprotein heamagglutinin and neuraminidase in their envelopes differentiates substantially the genus from each other. While the Morbiliviruses possess only haemagglutinin (N) in its surface, Rubulla virus/ Avulavirus possess both the H and N, while the Pneumoviruses possess neither of the two.

MEASLES VIRUS

Measles is the only human agent of the genus Morbillivirus. The measles virus is one of the most infectious viruses known and has been targeted by the World Health Organization for eradication.

Measles is monotypic, although small antigenic differences do occur between strains. The measles virus is relatively unstable at temperature higher than 40°C and pH below 5 and above 10. It is sensitive to ether and other organic solvents.

Source and Collection of Specimen

Measles virus can be easily isolated from blood, urine and nasopharyngeal washings. Blood sample must be collected within 4 days after the appearance of rash. The possibility of isolating the virus in the blood fast diminishes after 4 days of rash because of the development of neutralising antibody which begins to neutralise out the virus in the blood

Leucocytes must be separated from the whole blood as soon as the blood is collected. The leucocytes can be stored at -80°C for days before inoculation. The virus is present in the urine 14 days after rash and therefore provides an alternative to whole blood. The disadvantage of urine however is the lower titer and the toxicity effect on the cell. Before inoculation, urine must be diluted in one half volume.

Inoculation and Isolation

Measles virus can be isolated in primary cell lines such as primary African green monkey kidney, human embryonic kidney. Primary isolation can however be difficult and may require more than one passage before evidence of viral growth is observed. The discovery of the B95-8 cell line, an Epsein Barr transformed marmoset lymphocyte by Kobune and its adherent form B95a have made primary isolation of measles in cell culture simple. Recently, a novel cell line, the SLAM Vero-a genetically engineered cell line to which the co-receptor CD150 - the signaling lymphocytic activation molecule (SLAM) has been incorporated is now available in most laboratories for primary isolation of the virus. This is gradually replacing the B95a cell line because of its carcinogenic tendency. The separated leucocytes or lymphocytes can be co-cultured with the freshly trypnised cells or inoculated directly into the confluent monolayer. Urine specimen can be inoculated directly without further processing after the initial dilution..

Procedure

1. Prepare a monolayer of B95a in a 25 cm2 tissue culture flask in 10% DMEM or RPMI 1640.
2. After confluency, decant the medium and inoculate between 0.2 – 0.5 ml of the lymphocyte and incubate at 37°C for 1 hr.
3. Add about 10ml of 2% DMEM or RPMI 1640 and incubate further at 37oC.
4. Check daily for CPE.

If the virus is present, CPE will be observed within 36 hours. Measles CPE is characterised by syncythia with the appearance of multinucleated giant cells, appearance of stellate bodies and foamy type of CPE characterised by vacuoles and deposit of fat globules.

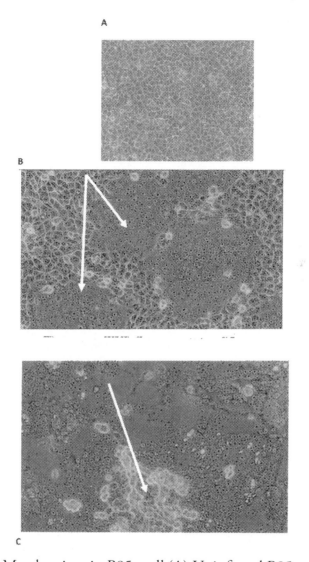

Fig 11.1 Measles virus in B95a cell.(A) Uninfected B95a cell line.
(B) Infected B95a cell line showing bulls eye type of CPE(arrow)
(C) Infected B95a cell line showing multinucleated giant
cells(arrow)

Measles forms good plaque under agar overlay and the method is
often used in virus neutralisation for antibody assay.

Virus Identification

For an experienced eye, the characteristic CPE of measles virus in cell culture guided by clinical symptoms can provide a presumptive identification of the virus. This must however be confirmed by other laboratory methods. Because measles virus is cell-associated, the immufluorescence staining technique provides a direct method of rapid virus identification. A good source of measles virus specific monoclonal antibody is available for this direct detection

Virus Neutralisation Test/ Plaque Reduction Neutralisation Test

Both the antibody neutralisation test, and the more accurate and sensitive plague reduction neutralisation test can be used to identify the virus. In both cases, known specific antibody (monoclonal) must be available. Since measles CPE develops slowly, a good virus and cell control must be set up to differentiate cell degeneration from CPE as long as the culture lasts.

PCR

A good PCR technique for the direct identification of the viral RNA is available. Good primers have been developed for this purpose.

IgM ELISA for Measles Identification

The IgM ELISA is the method recommended by the WHO for the Measles elimination/eradication programme for identification of the measles virus in infected children. This method has come to replace the conventional 4-fold antibody rise determination method using CFT or HI test.

Haemagglutination/Haemagglutination Inhibition Test

Measles HA/HI tests remain the most popular method in many laboratories for the identification of measles virus and for measuring antibody level following exposure or vaccination.

Measles antibody titre is relatively very low in tissue culture harvest. We now produce a high potent measles HA antigen in our lab in

Ibadan. Measles readily heamagglutinates African green monkey red blood cell and this property has been used for the identification of this virus. Again, a known specific measles virus antibody must be available.

PARAINFLUENZA VIRUSES

There are 4 serotypes of the human parainfluenza viruses – parainfluenza types 1, 2, 3 and 4. Parainfluenza viruses are the major causes of lower respiratory tract infection in infants and children as well as mild upper respiration disease in young adults. They have been associated with croup, pneumonia and broncholities.

Parainfluenza viruses share a lot in common with influenza viruses. However, one major difference between the two viruses is the non-segmented nature of the parainfluenza virus genome.

The parainfluenza viruses are distributed into 2 separate genera of the paramyxoviridae i.e. types: 1 and 3 belong to the Respirovirus genus while types 2 and 4 belong to the Rubulavirus. All the viruses are similar in appearance and biophysical characteristics. They all carry the glycoprotein heamagglutinin and neuraminidase in their surface envelopes. They are only differentiated by their antigenic reactivities.

Specimen Source and Collection

The specimens of choice for isolation of parainfluenza viruses are nasal or throat washings and pharyngeal swabs. Specimens should be collected in transport medium and transported to the laboratory cold. The chances of virus isolation are greater when the specimen is inoculated fresh without freezing.

Virus Inoculation and Isolation

Parainfluenza viruses are best isolated in primary cells lines. Primary simian, the LLC-MC2 or human kidney cell, Vero, African green monkey kidney and the human lung carcinoma cell line are all very sensitive for isolation. The cells must be treated with typsin-EDTA 1-5ug/mg for type 1 and 4 isolation (1-5 ug/mg). Virus isolation is better achieved when the cells are not maintained in calf serum.

Prior to inoculation, the maintaince medium should be poured off and washed with Hank's BSS. Inoculated cells should be incubated at 33°C.

There are no visible cytopathic effects in infected cells. Virus infection of the cultured cells can only be visualised by heamoadsorption or immunostaining with 0.5% fresh guinea pig rbc used to flood the surface of the infected cells. The red blood cells will adsorb to anywhere in the cell where viral replication has taken place. Virus infection of cells is characterised by syncytia formation which is more pronounced in types 2 and 3.

The procedure for the heamoadsorption method is as stated below:
Procedure
1. Decant the spent medium from the infected cell into a sterile tube.
2. Inoculate 0.2 ml of the 0.5% guinea pig rbc into the infected cell.
3. Incubate at 40C (parainfluenza 1, 2 and 3) or at 35 – 37°C (parainfluenza 4) for 20 minutes and make sure that the guinea pig rbc is in contact with the infected cells.
4. Pour off any unabsorbed rbc and wash the cell with cold PBS.
5. Observe the cells for evidence of viral growth which is evidenced by rbc attachment.
6. Fluids from cell showing positive haemoadsorption can be subcultured.

Virus Identification
Virus identification can be accomplished by a number of laboratory methods.

Direct Immunofluorescent Technique
Staining for rapid viral antigen detection utilises conjugated monoclonal antibody to any of the virus types for direct identification. This is done by detaching the cells from the tissue culture flask and suspending the

cell pellet in the spot well of the microscope slide. This is then stained with the type-specific monoclonal antibody conjugated to fluorescein. The slide can then be visualised under fluorescent microscope for flouroescence which is indicative of positive test.

Haemadsorption Inhibition Method
Parainfluenza viruses can be identified using the hemadsorption inhibition test. The hemadsorption method is a modified neutralisation test in which the indicator medium is the guinea pig rbc.

Procedure
1. Make a 10-fold dilution of the unknown virus and inoculate into three replicate tubes. After 3-5 days, add 0.2 ml of 0.5% guinea pig rbc. Calculate the hemadsorption end point.
2. Make a 2-fold dilution of the antiserum starting from 1:10.
3. Add equal volume of the antiserum to the virus containing 30-50 hemadsorption TCID 50 and mix well.
4. Allow mixture to stand at room temperature for 1 hour.
5. Inoculate double amount of mixture into 4 culture tubes per dilution.
6. Perform virus control by inoculating 0.1 ml of the virus dilution.
7. Incubate both control and test tubes at 33oC.
8. Three to five days later add 0.2 ml of 0.5% guinea pig RBC to each tube. Keep for 20 minutes and read the result.
9. Complete inhibition of hemadsorption by the parain-fluenza specific antiserum is considered as positive and indicates the identity of the virus.

PCR
Viral antigen can be detected in nasal secretions by the RT-PCR. A multiplex RT-PCR for the detection of types 1, 2, and 3 is available and is far more sensitive and rapid than the tissue culture method.

MUMPS VIRUS

The mumps virus belongs to the genus Rubulavirus of the Paramyxoviridae family.

The disease is characterised by parotitis i.e inflammation of the salivary glands presented in form of a swelling near the ear and a painful inflammation of the testes. The virus can also infect the central nervous system and other parenchymatous internal organs. Mumps virus and other related infections are responsible for about 20% of male sterility in Nigeria. (Osegbe and Amaku, 1985).

Source of Specimen and Collection

Saliva and throat swabs are the best sources for virus isolation. Saliva should be collected within the first 5 days after appearance of symptoms. Virus can also be isolated from the urine within 14 days after infections. Urine must be cleared of debris and concentrated by ultra centrifugation. About 15ml of urine should be centrifuged at 4°C for 10 minutes at 3500 rpm. After discarding the precipitate, the supernantant should be recentrifuged at 100,000g for 90 minutes in an ultra centrifuge. The precipitate can now be resuspended in 1 ml of cold PBS.

For patients with central nervous involvement, virus can be recovered from the CSF within 8-9 days after infection.

Specimens should be kept cold and inoculated immediately or kept at -70°C if immediate inoculation is not possible.

Virus Isolation and Identification

Mumps virus will grow in a variety of primary or established cell lines, like vero cell, primary monkey kidney and 8-9 day old embryonated eggs. Both the allantoic and amniotic cavity can be inoculated for virus isolation. Incubation is best at 37°C.

Mumps virus specific CPE is characterised by syncytia formation and lysis. Not all mumps virus strain will show CPE in cell culture. Further identification should be done by heamadsorption using guinea pig RBC.

The spot IF method can be used to detect the virus in infected cell using mumps virus specific monoclonal antibody. Allantoic and amniotic fluid should be tested for mumps virus heamagglutinating antigen 7 days after inoculation.

PCR

The RT-PCR provides a sensitive method for direct strain identification of the virus in clinical specimen, especially the CSF.

Serology

This is the method of choice for diagnosis since the virus grows slowly in tissue culture. A four fold or higher rise between the acute and convalescent phase sera using the HI, CFT, NT test is indicative of mumps virus infection. In the absence of paired sera, an ELISA technique comparing IgM and 1gG in acute phase sera will be appropriate. A higher IgM level is indicative of recent infection. A solid phase IgM capture ELISA is available.

RESPIRATORY SYNCYTIA VIRUS

Respiratory syncytia virus (RSV) is the major cause of paediatric respiratory viral infection in infants and young children although adults and the elderly are also susceptible to the virus. The virus is found in high titre in the upper respiratory tract as well as in nasal and throat washings collected in the early course of the infection.

RSV belongs to the family paramyxoviridae. It is enveloped and therefore it is easily inactivated by adverse environmental conditions like adverse heat, ether and other lipid solvents.

The virus is pleomorphic, spherical with a diameter of about 150-300nm. The disease is caused by the RSV and is characterized by fever and upper and lower respiratory tract symptoms like bronchiolitis and pneumonia.

Source of specimen and collection

The virus is best recovered from nasal and nasopharyngeal secretions or washing and nasal swabs. Specimens should be kept cold without freeze-thawing and should be inoculated into susceptible cell immediately.

Virus Inoculation and Isolation

Virus isolation in culture is the most definitive test. Respiratory syncytia virus will grow mainly in epithelial cells of human origin. Primary isolation is usually first attempted in human heteroploid cell lines like HEp-2, HeLa and A549 cells. The virus can also grow in other cell line like MRC-5. Syncytia cytopathic effect will be observed in positive cultures within 3 to 7 days or greater, but viral effect can be visualised even faster by immunofluorescence.

Virus Identification

Rapid/Direct Detection of Viral Antigen

The Direct Immunofluorescent test can be used to detect the virus both in infected tissue culture and exfoliated epithelia of the respiratory tract.

RT-PCR is the most sensitive and specific test for the detection of the viral RNA. The RT-PCR has a sensitivity and specificity of about 90% and is more useful for the detection of the virus in adult patients because of the low titre of the virus in adults.

Neutralisation test.

Confirmation of the virus is usually by neutralization of infectivity in tissue culture by a known RSV specific antiserum. The complement fixation test can also be used to detect the antigen.

Serology

An ELISA antigen capture technique is available for the detection of the virus antigen. ELISA can also detect antibody to the virus. Antibody detected by ELISA are usually higher in titre than those of CFT or neutraliSation test.

An RSV-specific antiserum conjugated to the enzyme or dye must however be available.

PARAMYXOVIRUSES OF VETERINARY IMPORTANCE

CANINE DISTEMPER VIRUS

Canine Distemper virus belongs to the genus Morbillivirus. The virus is the cause of measles – like disease in dogs characterized by gastroenteritis, pneumonitis, conjuctivitis and encepha-lomyelitis. The virus can cause disease in nearly all families of terrestrial carnivores.

The canine distemper virus is difficult to isolate. It takes days to weeks for the virus to grow. Confirmation of infection is by any of the following methods.

Immunofluorescent Detection of Distemper Inclusion Bodies
CDV inclusion bodies can be detected in the bladder, conjunctival membranes. Antibodies against CDV are coupled to fluorescein. The labelled antibody will combine with the virus in the affected organ to give a fluorescent colour. The presence of the inclusion body confirms distemper virus. However, non-detection of inclusion body does not rule out CDV infection.

IgM level in Acute Phase Sera
An ELISA technique that detects the level of IgM and IgG in acute phase sera can be used to detect the difference in the level of IgM and IgG. A higher IgM level than IgG is indicative of CDV infection. A modification of this test is the use of CSF for antibody detection. Result obtained is reliable because vaccine-induced IgM is ruled out.

Direct Detection of CDV RNA by PCR
The virus can be detected rapidly in clinical sample by the RT-PCR.

RINDERPEST VIRUS

Like canine distemper, Rinderpest virus is a morbillivirus of large cloven hoofed ruminants. It is a very important veterinary pathogen. The disease is characteriSed by severe gastroenteritis, inflammation, heamorrhage, necrosis and erosion of the gastrointestinal tract. The virus grows very well in lymphoid tissues and macrophages.

Rinderpest virus can be isolated in both primary and transformed cells for example Vero and bovine kidney (BK) cells.

Samples for virus collection are whole blood in heparin, conjuctival/lacrimal swabs, necrotic lesions, oral lesions, spleen, tonsil and lymph nodes. Specimens should not be frozen.

Virus identification can be through antigen detection using any of the following tests – Agar gel immunodiffusion, direct and indirect immunoperoxidase staining, counter immunoelectrophoresis and immuno fluorescent technique.

Viral RNA can be detected rapidly by the probe-hybridization technique or RT-PCR.

PESTES DES PETIT RUMINANTS (PPR)

PPR is a rinderpest-like disease of small ruminants i.e. goat and sheep. Goats are more susceptible to the virus. Clinical symptoms are similar to the symptoms of rinderpest in the large ruminants.

Samples for virus identification are the same as with rinderpest.

NEWCASTLE DISEASE VIRUS

The Newcastle disease virus is the only member of the genus Avulavirus, and it is the causative agent of an important disease of poultry, the Newcastle disease. The disease affects most species of birds both domestic and in the wild with high mortality. The disease is characterised by sneezing, nasal discharge and coughing and greenish diarrhea. The most stroking symptom is torticollis. Symptoms depend on the strain of the virus.

The virus can be isolated in 8 -10 day old embryonated eggs and primary chicken embryo fibroblast (CEF).

Cloacal swabs, tracheal swabs from living birds and lungs, kidney, liver, spleen and brain are the best sources of specimens for virus isolation.

Virus can be identified by the HI test using known specific monoclonal antibody.

The enzyme linked immunosorbent assay can also be used. PCR is used to detect viral RNA.

Further Reading

1. Chanock R, Parrott R. "Acute Respiratory Disease in Infancy and Childhood: Present Understanding and Prospects for Prevention. *Pediatrics* 1965; 36:21-39.

2. Glezen P, Denny FW. "Epidemiology of Acute Lower Respiration Disease in Children." *N Engl J Med 1959; 60: 731-738.*

3. Knipe. D.E. Lamb, R.A, Martin M.A., Roizman B. and Straus, S. Fields Virology 5th ed. Wolters Kluwer/Lippincott Williams and Wilkins.2007 Philadelphia, PA.

4. Osegbe, DN and Amaku, E.O. "The Causes of Infertility in 504 Consecutive Nigerian Patients." *International Urology and Nephrology 17: 4 1985.*

CHAPTER 12

Family ORTHOMYXOVIRIDAE
INFLUENZA VIRUSES

There are five genera under this family of which Influenza virus A, B, and C are the most important as far as human disease is concerned. Influenza virus has probably been associated with pandemics than any other virus in history. The evidence that avian influenza can be directly transmitted into humans has made influenza viruses a major global health threat.

There are 3 types of Influenza virus – Influenza A, B, and C. Influenza A virus is further divided into subtypes depending on the antigenecity of the HA and NA molecules. There are currently 16 HA subtypes (H1 - H16) and 9 NA subtypes (N1-N9). There are no antigenic subtypes for B and C. The orthomyxoviruses are single-stranded RNA viruses with segmented genomes. Influenza A and B have 8 segments of the RNA while C has seven. The RNA is enclosed in a lipoprotein envelope with two types of glycoprotein carrying spikes- the heamagglutinin (H) and the neuraminidase (N). Influenza C has a single glycoprotein with heamagglutinin and neuraminidase activities. Heamagglutinin mediates attachment to cellular receptors while neuraminidase cleaves sialic acid from the receptor of infected cells leading to virus release. Influenza A viruses are designated by the type of H and N antigens, for example H1N1, H5N1, H7N7 etc.

Influenza viruses are unique among the other RNA viruses in that they undergo some important changes that are of very significant epidemiologic importance. Examples of such are antigenic drift, antigenic shift, recombination and reassortment. Antigenic drift is a minor change in the H and N proteins due to point mutation. It is observed only in Influenza A and B. Antigenic shift is a major antigenic change in the H and N during which time a new H or N subtypes which is immunologically different from previous strains are evolved. It is caused by reassortment usually between human and avian viruses and/or direct transmission of avian or swine influenza viruses to human where they may establish transmission.

Source of Specimen and Collection

The preferred specimens for virus isolation are throat washing, throat swabs, and nasopharyngeal swabs. These must be collected within 24-48 hours. Autopsy tissues from lungs can also be collected.

Virus Inoculation and Isolation

Ten -11 day old embryonated chicken egg is still the best choice for Influenza virus isolation. The virus can be inoculated into either the allantoic or amniotic cavity with incubation at 33°C – 34°C.

Avian and equine strains are best isolated when inoculated into the allantoic cavity at 33°C – 37°C.

Recent human isolates are a bit more difficult to isolate in embryonated eggs. The growth of Influenza virus in embroyonated eggs most of the time gives rise to antigenic variants characterised by mutation in their H proteins (Burnet 1936).

Influenza A and B viruses can also be isolated in Madin-Darby canine kidney (MDCK) cell culture.

This cell will not support the growth of avian influenza virus. A visible CPE is not always observed in cell culture. The presence of virus is therefore recognized by hemoadsorption with guinea pig RBC.

Other primary cell lines of monkey, hamster, chicken kidney, chicken embryo fibroblast, primary human epithelia cells as well as Vero will support the growth of Influenza virus, but less efficiently than the MDCK.

Virus Identification

Haemagglutination inhibition test is the most commonly used method for initial identification of Influenza virus after isolation. Both guinea pig and chicken RBC can be used but Guinea pig RBC gives higher titre at primary isolation, the latter is agglutinated at a higher titre after passages for proper differentiation. Influenza virus specific antibody should be used.

Rapid Viral Diagnosis

A wide variety of rapid viral diagnoses are now available. The immunoflorescent spot technique using Type A or B monoclonal antibody can be used to detect the antigen. A negative FA does not always rule out influenza virus infection. Result should be confirmed by further culturing.

A new rapid assay based on the detection of neuraminidase activity is now available for Type A and B infections.

PCR

PCR has been used to detect Influenza virus RNA in respiratory samples.

Further Reading

1. Burnet F.M. "Influenza virus on the Developing Egg: Changes Associated with the Development of Egg Passage Strain of Virus." *Br. Journal of Exp Pathol 1936; 17: 282-293.*

2. Delong mo, Tran TT, Truong HK, al. "Oseltamivir Resistance During Treatment of Influenza A (H5NI) infection." *N Engl J Med 2005; 353; 2667-2672.*

3. Delorme L, Middleton Pj. "Influenza A Virus Associated with Acute Encephalopathy." *Am J Dis child 1979; 133:822-824.*

4. Knipe. D.E. Lamb, R.A, martin M.A., Roizman B. and Straus, S. Fields Virology 5th ed. Wolters Kluwer/ Lippincott Williams and Wilkins.2007 Philadelphia, PA.

CHAPTER 13

FAMILY REOVIRIDAE

There are 12 Genera within the family Reoviridae. They include vertebrate, arthropod and plant pathogens. Only three of these Genera-the Orbivirus, Reovirus and Rotavirus will be mentioned here. For further reading the reader is directed to Fields Virology (Knipe and Howley). Viruses in these genera share some common similarities. They are all double stranded RNA viruses having about 10, 11, or 12 double stranded RNA segments. Yet, they differ in their structure, physico-chemical properties, pathogenesis and epidemiology. Orbiviruses, unlike the Reovirus and Rotavirus, are arthropod-borne. Viruses of this family are non-enveloped.

ORBIVRIUSES

There are 21 sero groups of the genus Orbivirus. Within each serogroup, several serotypes can be identified by neutralisation test. Different orbiviruses infect a wide variety of vertebrate hosts, domesticated and wild. Notable among these are the Bluetongue disease virus of sheep, Epizootic haemorrhagic disease of deer and African horse sickness.

THE ORTHOREOVIRUSES

The Reoviruses comprise fusogenic and non-fusogenic reoviruses of mammals and birds. The fusogenic viruses are characterized by fusion of infected cells into giant multinucleated syncytia. Reovirus were initially isolated from human respiratory and enteric tracts, but were not associated with a definitive serious disease. The name reovirus which is an acronym of respiratory enteric orphan was derived from this initial characteristics of these viruses.

To differentiate the initial isolates of the reoviruses from the other members of the family which are often referred to in general as Reoviruses, the prefix – ortho – is attached. Orthoreoviruses are icosahedral in shape, with a double-layered capsid consisting of 92 capsomeres. The genome is made up of 10-12 segments of ds RNA. They are ether resistant as a result of the absence of a lipid envelope. There are four serotypes that can be identified by neutralisation and heamagglutination inhibition tests. Type 1 was first isolated from a healthy child (type 1 Lang). Type 2 (Type 2 Joan) was first isolated from a child presenting with diarrhea while Type 3 was initially isolated from children presenting with diarrhea (Type 3 Dearing) and upper respiratory infection(Type Abney). All the serotypes are capable of multiplying in a variety of cells of non primate origin including pig, calf, dog, cat, guinea pig and hamster cells where they induce characteristic CPE.

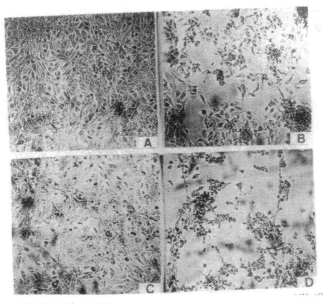

Fig. 13.1 CPE induced by Reovirus in non primate kidney cells.

A. Uninfected cat kidney
B. Cat kidney infected with type 1
C. Uninfected guinea pig kidney cell
D. Infected guinea pig kidney infected with type 1

Reproduced with permission- G.D. Hsiung. Diagnostic Virology, Yale University Press, 1982.

Although all ortho-reoviruses share a common group antigen that can be detected by complement fixation test, they can however be distinguished serologically into the three antigenic groups by the NT and H1 tests. Serotypes 1 and 2 agglutinate human group O-erythrocytes at high titre. Type 3 agglutinates bovine erythrocytes at 4°C. This can be used to differentiate type 3 from the other 2 serotypes.

Source of specimen and collection

Stool is the best and optimum specimen for virus isolation, but viruses can be isofrom throat swabs, nasal washing, CSF and urine. For initial isolation, primary kidney cells of primate and non-primate origin are susceptible.

Virus Inoculation and Isolation

Confluent monolayer cells should be inoculated with fresh specimen, not necessarily frozen. Inoculated cells must be incubated at 30-37°C. Reovirus CPE is characterised by cellular granulation, and not rounding. The CPE can easily be confused with the normal cell degeneration due to aging. A good control uninoculated cell should therefore be kept along for guidance. The more the number of passages of the virus isolates, the more definite and evident the CPE.

Virus Identification

Reovirus isolates can be identified by a variety of laboratory tests. Virus isolation remains the most important step towards identification. Initial identification can be based on the characteristic CPE.

Viral antigen detection

Detection of viral antigen in infected tissue or material can be accomplished by the direct immunofluorescent technique. An indirect Immunofluorescence with infected cell as target antigen can be used to detect antibody in the human serum. ELISA technique for the detection of antigen in tissue culture, as well as antibody detection in serum, is widely used in many clinical laboratories. Molecular technique such as in-situ and blot-dot hybridization and RT-PCR can be used for the detection for reovirus RNA and mRNA in infected cells.

Haemagglutination and Haemagglutination Inhibition tests

Reoviruses can be identified in HI test using human group O RBC. Usually tissue culture harvested fluid is a good source of the antigen. Agglutination takes place at temperature 4°C, 22°C and 37°C using 0.75% human group O RBC suspension in normal saline for types 1 and 2. Type 3 will only agglutinate bovine RBC under the same conditions.

Detection and identification of new serotypes can be achieved by a panel of type-specific antisera in HI. Sera must be pretreated and adsorbed with human group-O erythocytes. HI test result is best at 22°C

Plaque Reduction Neutralisation Test

Reoviruses produce good plaques when overlayed with agar medium in monkey kidney cells or guinea pig embryo cells. The plaque reduction neutralisation test (PRNT) can be used to identify new serotypes in the presence of panel of type specific antisera. Fetal bovine serum or skim milk must be used instead of calf serum in the medium because of the possible presence of reovirus antibody in calf serum.

Further Reading

1. Bangaru B, Morecki R, Cilaser JH, et al. "Comparative Studies of Biliary Atresia in Human newborn and

Reovirus- induced Cholangitis in Weanling Mice." *Lab invest 1980; 43; 456-462.*

2. Glaser JH, Balistreri WF, Morecki R. "Role of Reovirus Type 3 in Persistent Infantile Cholestasis." *J pediatr 11984;105: 912-915.*

3. Knipe. D.E. Lamb, R.A, Martin M.A., Roizman B. and Straus, S. Fields Virology 5th ed. Wolters Kluwer/Lippincott Williams and Wilkins.2007 Philadelphia, PA.

4. Morecki R, Glaser JH, Chos, et al. Biliary Artesia and Reovirus type 3 Infection. *New Eng J Med 1982;307 (8): 481-484.*

5. Richarrdson SC, Bishop RF, Smith AL. "Enzyme Iinked Immunosorbent Assays for Measurement of Reovirus immunoglobulinG, A, and M Levels in Serum." *J Clin Microbial 1988; 26(9: 111871-1873.*

6. Rosen L. "Reoviruses in Animals other than Man." *Ann NY Acad Sci 1962; 101:461-465.*

7. Sabin AB. Reoviruses. *"Science 1959; 1130;1389."*

8. Selb B Weber B. A Study of Human Reovirus IgG and IgA antiboclies by ELISA and Western Blot. *J Virol Meth 1994; 47(1-2):15-25.*

9. Stanley NF. "Reoviruses." Br Med Bull 1967:23:150-154

10. Tai JH, Williams JV, Edwards KM, et al. "Prevalence of Reovirus-specific Antibodies in Young Children in Nashville, Terressee." *J Infect Dis 2005; 191:1221-1224.*

ROTAVIRUSES

Rotaviruses infect humans and a variety of non-human species. They are the major cause of severe diarrhoea in infants and children and other non-human species like calves, piglets. The virus was first implicated in infantile diarrhea presenting with gastroenteritis. The group derives its name "rota" from the wheel-like structure of the virus. It is about 100 nm in diameter. It possesses a three-layered icosahedral capsid with 60 protein spikes extending from the smooth surface of the outer shell. It is a double stranded RNA virus with 11 segments of the viral RNA. The matured virus is non-enveloped.

There are multiple serogroups with multiple serotypes in the same sero-groups. Viruses of the same serogroups share cross-reacting antigens that can be detected by IF, ELISA, and IEM. There are a total of seven serogroups – A-G. Group A, B, and C infects both humans and animals. Group D, E, F, and G infect only animals. Some human rotaviruses have shown some antigenic relationship with rotaviruses for non-human species; especially antigenic crossings have been demonstrated between human rotaviruses and those isolated from calves, mice and monkeys.

Source of Specimens and Collection

Stool is the specimen of choice for Rotavirus isolation. Virus can also be detected in duodenal mucosa following biopsy.

Virus inoculation and isolation

Rotavirus can now be isolated with some degree of efficiency in primary monkey kidney cells and human embryonic kidney cells.

Virus Identification

Direct detection of virus or antigen in stool is the best choice. Detection is best carried out in stools in the 1st to 4th day after diarrhea, because diarrhea coincides with virus shedding.

Direct detection by electron microscopy (EM) and immunoelectron microscopy

The direct detection of rotavirus by EM is specific because of the distinctive morphology of the virus. It is the most rapid diagnostic method. The direct detection by EM is as follows:

Procedure
1. Prepare a 20% stool suspension in Hank's BSS with 0.5% BSA.
2. Centrifuge at 1000 x g for 30 minutes at 4oC.
3. Either stain the supernatant with phosphotungstate acid (PTA) and examine directly under the EM.
4. Or sediment pellet in distilled water, and after negative staining examine under EM.

5. Immunoelectron microscopy (IEM)
1.   Partially purified concentrated stool extract is mixed with the appropriate dilution of antiserum to Rotavirus.
2. Incubate for 1 hour at room temperature.

Apply mixture to EM grids.

Stain negatively with PTA solution and examine with EM.

Detection of Rotavirus in stool can also be achieved by other laboratory methods.

Detection of rotavirus in cell culture

It is possible to recover human rotavirus from stool in tissue culture using monkey kidney cells. Isolation of rotavirus in tissue culture has made determination of the serotypes by neutralisation assay possible. The IF can also be used to detect the virus in tissue culture.

Detection by ELISA

The direct and indirect ELISA has been used to detect rotavirus particles in stools. A confirmatory ELISA which makes use of serotype specific monoclonal antibody in a sandwitch procedure has been developed. It may be necessary to use several monoclonal antibodies directed at different epitopes of the same serotype because of the epitope polymorphism within a serotype.

Other virus detection methods like the counter immunoelectroosmophoresis, gel electrophoresis of the rotavirus RNA, reverse passive haemagglutination assay and latex agglutination can be used to detect rotaviruses in clinical specimens.

Molecular methods of detection

Rotavirus serotype can be determined by sequencing of either the VP4 or VP7 genes. RT-PCR is now used for genotyping positive-samples that cannot be typed by ELISA. In situ hybridization assay has also been developed. This method is highly specific and sensitive.

Serology

Serological response to rotavirus infection can be measured by IEM which is already described above, complement fixation text (CFT), IF, immune adherent heamaggltination assay, ELISA, neutralisation test and heamagglutination.

Further Reading

1. Bern C, Martines J, De zoysa I, et al. "The magnitude of the Global Problem of Diarrhoeal Disease; a Ten – year Update. *Bull WHO 1992; 70:705 – 714.*

2. Coulson BS, Kiokwood C. "Relation of VP7 Amino Acid Sequence to Monoclonal Antibody Neutralization of Rotavirus and Rotavirus Monotyoope. *J. Virol. 1991; 65:5968 – 5974.*

3. Fischer TK, Gentsh JR. Rotavirus Typing Methods and Algorithms Rev. *Med virol 2004; 14: 71-82.*

4. Parashar UD, Gibson CJ, Bresee JS, et al. "Rotavirus and Severe Childhood Diarrhea. *Emerg Infect Dis 2006; 12: 304 - 306.*

5. Parashar UD, Hummelman EA, Bresee JS, et al. "Global Illness and Deaths Caused by Rotavirus Disease in Children" *Emerg Infect Dis 2003; 9:565-572.*

CHAPTER 14

Family TOGAVIRIDAE

To the family Togaviridae belong some simple enveloped single stranded positive sense RNA viruses. Viruses belonging to the family were originally grouped into a large family of viruses including several arboviruses, but have recently been grouped into this separate family comprising two genera- the alphaviruses and the rubiviruses. There are many viruses under the alphaviruses, most of which are the causes of virus encephalitis worldwide. The genus Rubivirus is made up of a single member, the Rubella virus- the cause of a common childhood disease which is now being well controlled by a vaccine. Apart from the disease in children, rubella virus has been known to cause severe congenital defects in the fetus of infected women.

RUBELLA VIRUS

The rubella virus belongs to the genus Rubivirus of the Togaviridae family. Rubella virus is the aetiological agent of a predominantly childhood disease that is characterised by a low grade fever and mild upper respiratory symptoms in which the lymph nodes of the neck are enlarged. This is followed by generalised rash which may last for 2 to 3 days. The impact of rubella is however more felt in pregnant women in whom it can cause congenital abnormalities of the unborn infant, especially if the infection is contracted in the first trimester of the pregnancy. The virus can persist in the infant cells many months after birth giving rise to congenital rubella syndrome (CRS).

The rubella virus is a positive-sense RNA virus possessing a lipid envelope. It is sensitive to ether, chloroform and other lipid solvents. There is only one serotype of the rubella virus.

Source of Specimen and Collection

The best source of specimen for virus isolation is throat swabs and/or nasopharyngeal secretions. These specimens must be collected a week before and 2 weeks after the appearance of rash. Acute phase blood, cerebrospinal fluid (CSF), urine, amniotic fluid, placental and fetal tissues at time of birth are also good sources for virus isolation.

Virus Inoculation and Isolation

Rubella virus can be readily isolated in primary African green monkey kidney cells, BHK-21, RK13, and Vero cells. The RK-13 cell is preferable. The optimum temperature for virus isolation is at 35°C. Virus isolation can also be attempted in primary human cells, like human embryonic fibroblasts, human amniotic cells, where it may not demonstrate any visible cytopathological effect.

The virus will however show visible effect in BHK-21, RK-13 and Vero cells where it can grow to very high titre at optimum temperature of 35°C. CPE is characterized by rounding and detachment.CPE may be observed within 7 days or may require 2 or 3 serial blind passages.

Rubella virus forms clear and sharp plaques in RK13 and vero cells.

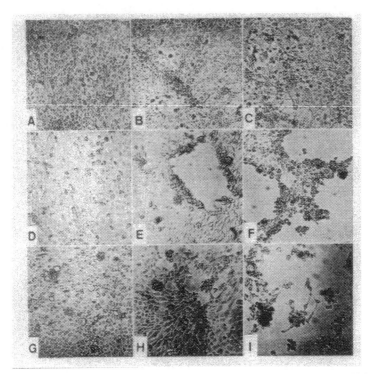

Fig. 14.1. CPE induced by rubella virus in rabbit kidney cell line.

A-C. RK-13 cultures (A)Uninoculated (B) 5 days (C) 8 days pi
D-F. RK1-H cultures (D) Uninoculated (E) 5 days (F) 8 days pi
G-I. RK1-FC cultures (G) Uninoculated (H) 5 days (I) 8 days pi
Reproduced with permission- G.D. Hsiung. Diagnostic Virology, Yale University Press, 1982.

Virus Identification

The clinical symptoms associated with rubella are such that can be easily confused with similar symptoms associated with maculo papular rash. Rubella must be differentiated from measles, human herpes virus 6 (roseola) and rash-associated enteroviruses, and parvovirus infection with which the symptoms are so similar. Rubella can also be confused with other flavivirus infections like Denge, West Nile, and Sindbis especially in endemic areas. Therefore final diagnosis of rubella requires laboratory identification.

Neutralisation test

This is the most specific test for the identification of rubella virus. The standard constant virus varying serum method of neutralization test method can be used.

Procedure
1. Titrate the virus suspension to determine the virus titre.
2. Calculate $100TCID50$ from the titre.
3. Make 2 serial dilution of a known rubella virus antiserum and add equal volume of the $100TCID50$ into each of the serum.
4. Incubate mixture of virus/serum at $37\,^{\circ}C$ for 1 hour.
5. Inoculate 0.2ml of each mixture into 4 culture tubes of RK13 and incubate at $35\,^{\circ}C$. Observe daily for CPE.
6. Neutralisation of infectivity will be observed in those tubes where the rubella antiserum is available to neutralise the virus. CPE will not be observed in such tubes.

Virus Interference assay

Identification of rubella virus can also be made using virus interference assay.

Rubella virus, when grown in GMK will not show visible CPE but when the same cell is inoculated with ECHO 11, CPE will be visible in the cells. However, a rubella infected cells will not show ECHO 11 CPE because of interference. This method is also used in the identification of rubella virus.

Procedure
1. Repeat steps 1-4 above.
2. Inoculate 0.2ml of each mixture into 3 or 4 tubes of GMK cells and incubate at $35\,^{\circ}C$.
3. At day 7, add $1000TCD50$ of ECHO 11 into each of the tube and observe for CPE.
4. In tubes where the rubella virus was neutralised by the rubella antisera, ECHO 11 CPE will be observed.

Rubella IgG Avidity Tests

1. Rubella reinfection can occur, especially in those whose immunity was induced by vaccination rather than by natural infection. However, reinfection by rubella during the first trimester of pregnancy is thought to pose minimal risks to the fetus but cases of CRS arising from rubella reinfection have often been reported. Therefore, it is important to distinguish reinfection from primary infection by rubella during the first trimester of pregnancy. One solution for the differentiation of primary from reinfection could be the measurement of the antigen-binding avidity of specific IgG. The avidity of IgG is low after primary antigenic challenge but matures slowly within weeks and months.

Procedure

This is a radial immunodifussion test and it is semi-quantitave.

1. Pour into a petri dish molten agar to which a known concentration of the rubella antigen has been mixed.
2. Punch antibody wells in the antigen-laden agar and fill the wells with dilutions of the different sera from the patient.
3. Flood the agar with 0.8% day-old chicken RBC.
4. Incubate overnight at 40C °r at 370C ᶠor one to two hours.
5. Observe and assess the type of zone of haemolysis around the antibody wells.

Haemolytic zones with soft diffuse outer margins are produced by antibodies of low avidity. Haemolytic zones with discrete outer margins are produced by antibodies of high avidity. Zones that were neither diffuse nor discrete are classified as equivocal.

Heamagglutination Inhibition Test

Rubella virus demonstrates heamagglutination activity when used against 0.5% day old chicks, adult goose or pigeon RBC in PBS. HA antigen can be extracted from infected cells or supernantant virus using Tween 80 and ether.

Procedure
1. Determine the HA titer of the rubella virus using 0.5% of the day old chick, or adult goose or pigeon RBC.
2. Treat the serum by inactivating at 56 °C for 30 minutes. Remove non-specific lipoprotein inhibitor and non-specific agglutinins with kaolin and chick RBC respectively.
3. Make a two-fold dilution of the serum starting from 1:2.
4. Add 4 HA units of the rubella antigen in equal volume to the diluted serum and incubate at 4 °C or 22°C.
5. Add 50ul of the chick RBC and again incubate at either 22 °C or 4 °C.
6. Read the result.

The dilution of the serum showing complete inhibition of the haemagglutination of the 4 HA unit of the rubella virus is the titre of serum.

HI antibody of 1:8-1:10 is evidence of rubella virus immunity.

Further Reading
1. Hsiung GD, Caroline KY, Fong and Marie L. Landry. *Hsiung's Diagnostic Virology* 4th ed. Yale University Press 1994.
2. Knipe. D.E. Lamb, R.A, Martin M.A., Roizman B. and Straus, S. *Fields Virology* 5th ed. Wolters Kluwer/Lippincott Williams and Wilkins.2007 Philadelphia, PA.
3. Zimmerman L, Ree F.S. "Rubella: UPD Surveillance Manual" published by CDC (Attanta) 2003:1-12.

CHAPTER 15

Family RHABDOVIRIDAE

About 185 different viruses isolated from animals, birds and plants make up the family Rhabdoviridae. Prominent among them are the Rabies virus, Lagos bat virus, Mokola virus, Divenhage virus, all belonging to the Lyssavirus genus. Of particular veterinary importance are the vesicular-stomatistis virus (VSV) and the Bovine ephemeral fever virus belonging to the Vesiculovirus and Ephemerovirus genera respectively.

The viruses are differentiated from all other enveloped single stranded RNA virus with which they share a lot in common by their elongated bullet shaped morphology.

RABIES VIRUS

Rabies is one of the oldest infectious diseases. The virus is transmitted usually by infected dogs or other canines and bats although some non-bite exposures have been reported. The outcome is almost always fatal after manifestation of clinical symptoms.

The incubation period in rabies is variable, may be as short as weeks and as long as many years. Manifestation of clinical symptoms often depends on how far the site of the bite is far from the central nervous system. The disease is characterised in man by photophobia, hydrophobia, musculoskeletal pain, anxiety, agitation, dysphagia, hypersalivation, paralysis and delirium. Clinical symptoms in dogs is like in human but characterised by loss of fear for humans.

Specimen source and sample collection

The best sources of specimen are saliva, brain stem and other infected tissues. Ante-mortem skin biopsies can be collected from the occipital position of the neck.

Post-mortem samples are the brain, central nervous system, specifically the brain stem or hippocampus.

Virus inoculation and isolation

Rabies virus can be easily isolated in tissue culture. A 10% suspension of rabies virus containing specimen from saliva or brain inoculated into Vero cells, HEp-2 or neuroblastoma cells will yield virus. CPE will appear in positive samples within the first 7 days.

Rabies virus can also be isolated in 1-2 day old mice when inoculated intracerebrally.

Virus identification

Rabies virus can be identified in post-mortem tissue, tissue culture or mouse-brain by the direct immunofluorescent (IFT) technique. However, a rabies specific fluorescein conjugated antibody must be used.

The avidin-biotin immunohistochemical staining of intracytoplasmic inclusion in the neuron is specific for virus identification.

Direct Giemsa staining for the characteristic Negri bodies in the hippocampus of the brain has been used for virus identification for a long time.

Direct examination of corneal smear impressions by the immunofluorescent antibody techniques is used for both human and animal specimen.

RT-PCR

Rabies virus specific RNA can be detected by the RT-PCR. RT-PCR can be used for direct amplification of the rabies virus from saliva and brains while sequencing is used to identify variants.

Serology

Virus neutralising antibodies can be detected by the neutralisation test (NT). This is particularly useful in dogs to determine immunity following vaccination.

Further Reading

1. Baer G.M. Pathogenesis to the central nervous system: In Baer G.M . ed. The natural history of Rabies; New York: Academic Press; 1975; 181 – 198.
2. Leach CN, Johnson H.N. "Human Rabies, with Special Reference to Virus Distribution and Titre." *Am J. Trop Med 1940; 20:335-340.*
3. Knipe. D.E. Lamb, R.A, Martin M.A., Roizman B. and Straus, S. *Fields Virology* 5th ed. Wolters Kluwer/Lippincott Williams and Wilkins.2007 Philadelphia, PA.

CHAPTER 16

Family FILOVIRIDAE

The Filoviruses are a large group of enveloped viruses with non-segmented negative strand RNA molecules. The unique structure of the Filoviruses necessitated its being grouped in a separate family, Filoviridae. Two important viruses – the Marburg virus and the Ebola virus constitute two separate genera in the family i.e. the Marburgvirus and the Ebolavirus. There is only one specie of the Marburg virus while there are four separate species of the Ebola virus namely Zaire ebolavirus, Sudan ebolavirus, Reston ebolavirus and Ivory Coast ebolavirus. Both viruses are classified as heamorrhagic fever viruses because of their high mortality and explosive nature of outbreak and pathological damage observed in infected patients.

Marburg heamorrhagic fever was first reported among three laboratory workers in Marburg, Germany after handling tissue cultures from monkeys imported from Uganda.

The first cases of Ebola heamorrhagic fever were reported in the old Zaire and Sudan in 1976. Both the Marburg and the Ebola viruses constitute very important source of laboratory and hospital infections.

The filoviruses are pleomorphic in structure with distinct bacilliform or filamentous forms which can either be U shaped or elongated or circular with length ranging between 790-1,200nm. The filamentous form can be as long as 14,000nm.

The virion is helical with a diameter of 80nm. Marburg and Ebola heamorrhagic fevers are very severe and characterizsed by acute haemorrhages which include petechiae, ecchymoses, uncontrolled oozing from venipunctured sites, mucosal heamorrhages and visceral effusions involving gastrointestinal, respiratory vascular and neurologic systemic manifestations.

Specimen source and sample collection

Because of the very virulent nature of these viruses and the ease of person to person transmission, the viruses are best handled in a "Class 4" maximum containment biosafety cabinet. BSL-4.

Specimens suspected to be those of Marburg and Ebola viruses must be transported to these laboratories that are capable of handling them. Specimens must be transported with maximum security in accordance with IATA regulations.

During sample collection, adequate care must be taken to reduce possibility of infection through barrier nursing, avoidance of needle pricking and immediate disposal of contaminated materials.

Specimens to be collected include serum, whole blood and tissues especially the liver. Blood for viral antigen detection must be collected within 3-16 days after the onset.

Virus handling and inoculation

All samples for virus detection should be rendered non infectious by treatment with Gamma irradiation, chemicals, exposure to Colbalt 60 and treatment with guanidinium isothiocyanate. After such treatment, samples can be handled outside the BSC4. Samples for virus isolation such as serum must be handled inside the BSC-4 containment.

Virus isolation

Filoviruses grow in a large number of cells. However, Vero and Vero E6 are the best.

CPE may not be observed for primary isolation. Repeated passages may yield CPE. Inoculation into guinea pig will produce fatal outcome after some passages.

Virus identification

Antigen Detection: Viral antigen detection can be done by ELISA.
Antibody Detection: The direct IgG and IgM, and the IgM Capture
ELISAs are used to detect the antibody in serum. Because filovirus
patients often die within a short time, there may not be time for
seroconversion.

RT-PCR - very useful for making diagnosis during the acute phase. RT-
PCR will detect the virus RNA in blood or serum as well as tissues.

Serology

The indirect IF techniques can be used for screening while Immunoblot
is used to confirm.

Test	Target	Source	Remarks
IFA	Antibodies	Serum	Rapid and simple
ELISA	Antibodies	Serum	Rapid, specific sensitive
Immunoblot	Antibodies	Serum	Protein specific Interpretation often difficult
Antigen Detection ELISA	Antigen	Blood, Serum tissues	Rapid and sensitive
Immunohistochemistry	Antigen	Tissue (skin liver)	Slow material inactivated
Fluorescence Assay	Antigen	Tissue, liver	Rapid Easy
PCR	Viral Nucleic Acid	Blood, Serum Tissue	Rapid and sensitive
Virus Isolation	Viral particle	Blood, tissue	Slow. Virus isolates available for studies

Table 16.1 Laboratory assays used for the diagnosis of Filoviruses

Further Reading
1. Hugo Caldas. "Filoviridae: Ebola and Marburg Viruses."
   Honour School of life Sciences. 1997-98.
2. Knipe. D.E. Lamb, R.A, Martin M.A., Roizman B. and
   Straus, S. Fields. *Virology* 5th ed. Wolters Kluwer/Lippincott
   Williams and Wilkins.2007 Philadelphia, PA.

CHAPTER 17

Family FLAVIVIRIDAE

The family Flaviviridae consists of three genera, the Flavivirus, Pestivirus and Hepacivirus. Only the Flavivirus will be described here. (see Chapter 21 for Hepatitis C virus).

The Flaviviruses comprise more than 70 viruses many of which are arthropod-borne human pathogens (Arboviruses). They cause many types of diseases varying from fever, encephalitis and haemorrhagic fevers. Such diseases include yellow fever, dengue haemorrhagic fever, dengue shock syndrome, Japanese encephalitis, West Nile, St Louis encephalitis, tick borne encephalitis, and Murray Valley encephalitis.

The flaviviruses are small RNA viruses with a lipid bilayer envelope. On the surface of the virion are two major proteins, the E-protein which is the envelope protein and the M-protein, the membrane protein. They surround a nucleocapsid of single-stranded positive sense genome. The flaviviruses are categorised into antigenic complexes based on serological criteria. The flaviviruses share some physicochemical properties among themselves. They are ether-sensitive and contain a small icosahedra nucleocapsid. They replicate in the cytoplasm and acquire the envelope during budding. As arboviruses, most members of the flaviviruses have an arthropod as vectors usually mosquitoes and ticks. The viruses can be biologically transmitted by such vectors.

YELLOW FEVER VIRUS

Yellow fever virus is the prototype of the Flavivirus genus. It was the first filterable human disease causing agent discovered. The virus is transmitted by different species of mosquitoes.

The disease is characterised by an incubation period of 3-6 days or as long as 14 days, which may be followed by clinical symptoms of fever, chills, headache muscle pain, nausea and vomiting, haemorrhages, epitasis and jaundice.

Source of specimen and collections

Serum is the best source for virus isolation. The liver and brain provide good sources of specimen after death. Serum must be collected within the first 4 days after onset. Virus can be isolated from the liver 14 days after the appearance of clinical symptoms. Pooled trapped mosquitoes also provide a good source for virus isolation.

Virus inoculation and isolation

Yellow fever virus is easily isolated in 1-2 day old mice. Inoculation is intracerebrally with $0.01 - 0.02$ml of viral suspension. Serum for virus inoculation may be inoculated undiluted in medium containing 5% fetal bovine serum (FBS) or diluted with medium up to 10^{-3}. Yellow fever virus can also be isolated in Toxorhynchites or Aedes species of mosquitoes when inoculated intrathoracically. This method requires some expertise.

Tissue Culture: Various cell lines such as Vero, HEp-2, BHK- 21 or the mosquito cell line from the pseudoscutellaris will permit the growth of YFV. Undiluted serum, 10% brain and liver suspensions and pooled mosquito suspensions made in medium containing 20% FBS and clarified by medium speed centrifugation (8-12,000g for 30 minutes can be inoculated into these cell lines.

Virus Identification

Mouse average survival time (AST)

Pathogenecity of YF for mice can be used for initial presumptive identification of the virus. The AST of most arbovirus, especially

YFV is between 5-6 days depending on the initial titre of the virus. The AST can be calculated as follows:

Procedure
1. Inoculate intracerebrally 0.01-0.02 ml of viral suspension into six 1-4 days old mice.
2. Examine the mice daily for hind limb paralysis or death.
3. Record paralysis or death.
4. Calculate the average survival times of mice.
5. The AST= $\frac{\text{Sum of animals that survived each day}}{\text{Number of days the experiment lasted}}$

Brains from dead mice or those showing signs should be inoculated i/c into another group of mice for confirmation by serology.

Antigen antibody detection
The IgM-antigen capture ELISA is a sensitive antigenic method for identification of YFV in serum or tissue. An enzyme-labelled species specific antibody must however be available.
The Immunofluorescent techniques can be used to detect virus antigen in the infected liver, cell culture and mosquitoes. A smear in a glass slide is made and stained with a fluorescein labelled antibody.

PCR
PCR is highly sensitive for early detection of yellow fever virus. Primers are available for the performance of such tests.

Serology
Serological methods for identification of YF virus include CFT, HI, NT, single radial heamolysis, indirect IF, ELISA. The CFT is specifically very good for detecting cross reactions since most of the flaviviruses share a common group antigen. Before ELISA became available, CFT was used for IgM antibody detection as a sign of recent infection. Since IgM disappears much more rapidly than IgG in serum the CFT is often more useful in detecting early infection.

The NT will detect both IgM and IgG and therefore is useful in monitoring past exposure to the virus or immunisation.

All these tests have been described in detail in their respective chapters in Section 2. Preparation of acetone extracted YF antigen from brain is described below.

Paired acute and convalescent sera are normally used for antibody detections, and are required to establish the diagnosis by rise in antibody titre. A 4-fold or greater rise or fall in antibody titre to the virus identifies the antibody as related to the virus. Because of extensive cross-reactivity among the flaviviruses, especially after secondary infection with heterologous strains, diagnosis is often complicated. Therefore, a suitable antigen must be available and the appropriate test used. The IgM capture ELISA is specific for most of the flaviviruses in both primary and secondary infections.

The laboratory diagnosis of other flaviviruses is similar to that of YFV. The interested reader is therefore referred for further reading on the specific flavivirus.

Mouse protection neutralization Test

Using a known positive YFV antiserum, mouse protection neutralisation can be done to identify YFV.

Procedure
1. Mix equal amount of YFV positive antiserum with a challenge virus.
2. Allow to incubate for 2 hours at 37oC.
3. Titrate the mixture in mice.
4. Simultaneously titrate the YFV alone.
5. Calculate the neutralisation index (NI) which is the difference between the virus/serum and virus alone.

An NI equal to or greater than 1 identifies the virus as YFV.

Plague reduction neutralisation test

The PRNT is another serological method for identification of YFV. An 80% or greater reduction in the number of plaques by the YFV specific antiserum identifies the virus as yellow fever virus.

Preparation of Sucrose acetone extracted antigen from mouse brain

Procedure
1. Infect a group of 1-4 day old mice with the YF virus through intracerebral inoculation.
2. Examine for paralysis or death.
3. Remove the brains with a sterile 18 inch gauge needle from the dead or fatally sick mice and weigh.
4. Homogenise for 1 minute in a blender by adding 4 volumes of cold 8.5% sucrose in distilled water.
5. Rapidly add 1 volume of the homogenate into 20 volumes of chilled acetone. Use a large syringe.
6. Shake vigorously. You may use an orbital shaker if available. Allow tissue to settle for 10-30 minutes at 4°C.
7. Gently aspirate the supernatant and discard. To the precipitate add the same volume of chilled acetone as in Step 5.
8. Again shake vigorously and allow the residue to settle at 4oC ʰor 60 minutes.
9. Discard the supernatant, and add a small amount of fresh acetone to the precipitate. This will remove the extracted tissue.
10. Transfer the sediment to a 15ml centrifuge tube and immersed in an ice bath. Vacuum dry for 2-3 hours.
11. The dried antigen is then rehydrated with borate buffered saline pH9.0 in volume equal to 0.004% of the original volume of the homogenate.
12. This antigen can be used for the haemagglutination inhibition test for identification of the virus.
13. Further inactivation of the antigen to eliminate any residual infective virus can be done by the addition of 10% beta-propiolactone (BPL) in cold PBS at a final concentration of 0.1% - 0.3% while stirring in a shelter for 72 hours at 4°C.

14. Test the antigen for the HA units.Goose red blood cells is normally used for YF HA, while inhibitors are removed by acetone treatment.

Reagents for YFV HI
Borate-Buffered Saline pH 9.0.

1.5M NaCl	-	80ml
0.05M H_3BO_3	-	100ml
1M NaOH	-	23ml
Distilled H2O	-	To make a litre

Adjust the pH as indicated below as shown in Table 17.1.

Dextrose Gelatin Veronal

Veronal	0.58gm
Gelatin	0.60gm
$CaCl_2$	0.02gm
Sodium veronal	0.38gm
$MgSO_4$-$7H_2O$	0.12gm
NaCl	8.5gm
Dextrose	10gm
Distilled H_2O	1000ml

Dissolve both the gelatin and veronal in water by heating and add the other reagents and mix. Sterilise by autoclaving at 10 lbs/in² for 10 minutes.

Further Reading

1. Karabatsos, N. *Supplement to the International Catalogue of Arboviruses. American of Trop med. Hyg 27; 1978.*
2. Knipe. D.E. Lamb, R.A, Martin M.A., Roizman B. and Straus, S. *Fields Virology* 5th ed. Wolters Kluwer/Lippincott Williams and Wilkins.2007 Philadelphia, PA.
3. Lanciotti R.S. "Molecular Amplification Assays for the Detection of Flaviviruses." *Adv Virus Res. 203; 61: 67-99.*

4. Monath. T.P. ed. St Louis Encephalitis. Washington D.C. American Public Health Association. 1980.
5. Theiler. M and Downs W.G. *The anthropod-borne Viruses of Vertebrates: An Account of the Rockefeller Foundation Virus Program.* 1951-1970. New Haven, Yale University Press 1973.

Solution A 0.15M NaCl, 0.2M Na₂HPO₄	Solution B 0.15M NaCl, 0.2M NaH₂PO₄	pH
3	97.0	5.75
12.5	87.5	6.0
22.0	78.0	6.2
32	68.0	6.4
45	55.0	6.6
55	45	6.8
64	36.0	7.0
72	28.0	7.2
79	21.0	7.4

Table 17.1 Adjusting the pH for yellow fever virus HI reagent

DENGUE HAEMORRHAGIC FEVER VIRUS

About one-third of the world's population lives in areas at risk for transmission of dengue virus infection. The disease is fast becoming a leading cause of illness and death in the tropics and subtropics where as many as 100 million people are infected yearly. Dengue fever (DF) is caused by any of four closely related viruses or serotypes: dengue 1-4. (DENV 1, DENV 2, DENV 3, DENV 4), Infection with one serotype does not protect against the others and sequential infections put people at greater risk for dengue heamorraghic fever (DHF) and dengue shock syndrome (DSS). There are no vaccines yet to prevent infection with dengue virus (DENV) and the most effective protective measures are those that avoid mosquito bites. *Aedes aegypti* is the principal mosquito vector of dengue viruses but *Aedes albopictus* will also transmit the virus.

The mosquito is closely associated with humans and their dwellings.

Dengue is characterised by an acute febrile illness accompanied by headache, retroorbital pain, body pain, often a rash, and other variable symptoms that can include frank or mild heamorrhagic manifestations (such as a petechial rash) or heamoconcentration, shock or coma.

Specimen source and sample collection

Blood (serum) is the best source of specimen. The blood must be collected at the acute stage and frozen for transportation to the laboratory. A second blood sample should be taken 6 or more days after appearance of symptoms.

Autopsy tissues are also sources for virus isolation.

Type of sample	Interval since the onset of symptoms	Type of Analysis
Acute Phase	Until 5 days	PCR
Covalescent	6 or more days	Serology(ELISA)

Table 17.2 Type of sample and analysis for Dengue fever diagnosis

Samples taken on days 4 and 5 of illness will yield very low titre virus and antibodies.

Virus inoculation and isolation

Dengue virus can be isolated in a variety of primary and continuous cell lines. The virus will grow very well in HL-CZ, a cell line of human origin derived from the promonocyte. The virus will also grow in LLC a cell line of monkey origin, MK2 , Vero, primary monkey kidney, BHK-21, mosquito cell lines C6/36 and AP 61.

The virus can be easily isolated in suckling mice and hamsters when inoculated intracerebrally.

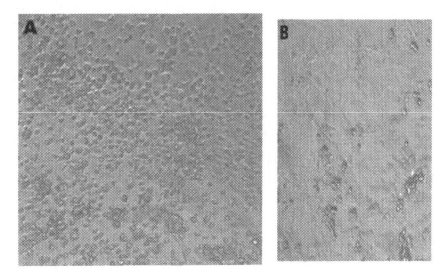

Fig 17.1 An infected LLC-MK2 cell line (A) showing CPE 6 day post infection. (B). Uninfected cell control.

Virus identification

Plaque Neutralisation Test

The serotype can be identified by the Plaque Reduction Neutralisation Test. However, a known positive monoclonal antibody to the serotype must be available to perfrom the test. An 80% or more reduction in plaque identifies the virus.

MAC ELISA

Immune response following a dengue virus infection produces IgM and IgG antibodies primarily directed against the virus envelope proteins. Anti–dengue IgM can be detected after the 6th or more days using the IgM Capture ELISA(MAC- ELISA). IgM antibodies for dengue remain elevated for 2 to 3 months after the illness. Because of this, the elevated IgM could be the result of an infection that occurred 2 to 3 months ago. MAC-ELISA has become an important tool for routine dengue diagnosis. MAC-ELISA has a sensitivity and specificity of approximately 90% and 98%, respectively but only when used five or more days after onset of fever (i.e. in convalescent phase).

IgG ELISA

The classic IgG ELISA used for the detection of a past dengue infection utilises the same antigens as the MAC ELISA. The assay is usually performed with multiple dilutions of the sera tested to determine an end-point dilution. This assay correlates with the hemagglutination inhibition assay (HI) previously used. A fourfold or greater increase in IgG antibody titers in paired (acute and convalescent) serum specimens also identifies the virus.

Immunofluorecent Test

Dengue virus can be identified during the acute phase infections by the identification of dengue viral antigen or RNA in autopsy tissue specimens by immunofluorescence or immunohistochemical analysis.

Molecular methods

RT-PCR

Specific dengue virus genome can be identified by reverse transcription-polymerase chain reaction (RT-PCR) from serum or plasma, cerebrospinal fluid, or autopsy tissue specimens during an acute febrile illness. Other molecular methods like one-step, real time RT-PCR or nested RT–PCR are now widely used to detect dengue viral genes in acute-phase serum samples. The detection of the dengue genome coincides with the viremia and the febrile phase of the illness.

Further Reading

1. Calisher C.H, Karabatsos N., Dalrymple J.M et al. "Antigenic Relationship Among Flaviviruses as Determined by Cross Neutralisation Tests with Polyclpnal Antisera. *Gen Virology.* 70:17-43.

2. Deubel V., Kinney R.M., Trem DW. "Nucleotide sequence and deduced amino acid sequence of the non-structural proteins of dengue type 2 virus, Jamaican genotype: Comparative analysis of the full length genome." *Virology 1988*; 165: 234-244.

3. Knipe. D.E. Lamb, R.A, Martin M.A., Roizman B. and Straus, S. *Fields Virology* 5th ed. Wolters Kluwer/Lippincott Williams and Wilkins.2007 Philadelphia, PA.

4. Russell P.K., McCown J.M. "Comparison of Dengue 2 and Dengue 3 Virus Strains by Neutralisation and Identification of Subtype Dengue 3." *Am of Trop med Hyg 1972;21:97-99.*

CHAPTER 18

Family RETROVIRIDAE

Viruses belonging to the family Retroviridae are different from other viruses because of their unique method of replication. The virion particles contain a genomic RNA which on entry to their host is reverse transcribed into a DNA form by the enzyme reverse transcriptase which is integrated into the chromosomal DNA of the host to form a provirus.

The Retrovirus comprises a large group of viruses found in vertebrates. They are grouped into 7 groups – Alpharetrovirus, Betaretrovirus, Gamma retrovirus, Delta retrovirus, Epsilon retrovirus, Lentivirus and Spumavirus. (Only the Lentivirus will be described here).

The Lentivirus consists of seven important viruses of which the human immunodeficiency virus 1 and 2 (HIV 1 & 2) are the most important. Others are simian immunodeficiency virus (SIV), equine infectious anaemia (EIAV), feline immunodeficiency virus (FIV), caprine arthritis encephalitis virus (CAEV) aNd Visna maedi virus.

THE HUMAN IMMUNODEFICIENCY VIRUS (HIV)

The Human Immunodeficiency Virus (HIV) is the causative agent of the Acquired Immunodeficiency Syndrome (AIDS). The disease was first recognised as a clinical entity in 1981. Within a space of two and half decades, it has acquired a world-wide pandemic and the major cause of death in individuals aged between 25 to 44 years.

This syndrome is characterised by generalised lymphadenopathy, opportunistic infections and a variety of uncommon cancers and a general depletion of CD4 + T-lymphocyte subset in the peripheral blood.

The HIV-1 was first isolated in 1983. A second HIV with distribution limited to a few West African states was discovered in very much later and named HIV-2 to distinguish it from the HIV-1.

The HIV-1 contains three major structural proteins – the Gag, Pol and Env proteins. The precursor proteins from the primary translation products give rise to the various functional proteins that become very important in the diagnosis and identification of this virus and in predicting the outcome of disease progression.

The Gag precursor pr55 Gag is cleaved into the Matrix protein p17, capsid protein p24, nucleocapsid protein p7 and p6. A combination of the Gag/Pol precursor, Pr 160, gives rise to protease protein p10, the heterodimeric RT (the p51), p66 and the integrase precursor p32. The third and very important primary structural precursor protein, the Env precursor gp160 is cleaved into surface protein gp120 and the trans membrane gp 41. The remaining regulatory and ancillary proteins – tat, rev, nef, vif, Vpr and Vpu perform various other functions.

Specimen source and sample collection

HIV-1 or 2 can be detected in most of the body fluids. However, blood, serum, semen and milk are the preferred clinical samples. Antibodies to HIV can be detected in the serum within 6-12 weeks of infection in most infected persons and virtually in all individuals 6 months after exposure.

Virus Isolation

Virus isolation is not usually necessary for diagnosis but becomes necessary to determine genotypes, strains and the various variants.

The virus can be isolated in mitogen-activated human peripheral blood mononuclear cells (PBMC). The virus can also be isolated in CD4+ T leukemia cells lines such as CEM, Jurkat, and Hut 78. Cytopathic effect on these cell lines may either be slow giving rise to low yield of the virus or may be rapid yielding very high titre of the virus. Some may induce syncytia when the infected PBMC is co-cultured with M-2 cell.

All HIV-1 strains can productively infect activated PBMC, some will replicate in cultures of monocyte derived macrophages. These strains are referred to as M-tropic strains. Isolates recovered late in the infection will grow very well in CD4$^+$ T cell lines. These strains are called T-tropic.

Virus Identification

Detection of the various products of the viral proteins and genes forms the basis of HIV-1 and 2 identification.

Enzyme-Linked Immunosorbent Assay (ELISA)

Laboratory diagnosis of HIV infection is usually made by detection of HIV-1 or -2 antibodies in serum. This test is used for initial screening. Many commercial ELISA kits are available, the principles of which are based on antigen antibody complex being detected by an enzyme indicator conjugated to a known positive antigen or antibody.

Besides the standard HIV ELISA, there are many commercial rapid tests available in the market. The advantage of these is the simplicity and wide range of operating temperatures which make them well-suited for use in point of care testing.

Confirmatory Test

Positive or reactive sera in the screening tests are subjected to confirmatory test to detect antibodies to the various HIV antigens. This is done by the Western Blot.

Western Blot Method

The HIV Western Blot consists of a thin cellulose strip in which the various important HIV -1 or 2 proteins have been embedded. As a confirmatory test, the Western Blot is used to identify the presence of the various antibodies to the HIV proteins (Fig 18.1).Thus the presence of HIV antibodies in a given serum will be determined by their reactivity with the antigens that have been embedded and separated by their molecular weights in the strip. The HIV proteins are as follows:

ENV	gp^{160}
	gp^{120}
	gp^{41}
POL	p^{68}
	p^{53}
	p^{32}
GAG	p^{55}
	p^{40}
	p^{24}
	p^{18}

Different commercial kits are now available to which all the above HIV antigens have been electrophorectically immobilised.

Procedure
1. Take out the strip and allow to equilibrate at room temperature.
2. Add serum from the patient to be tested to the strip.
3. Incubate at 37^0C for 1 hr to allow antigen antibody reaction to take place. If antibody or antibodies are present, specific bands to the HIV antigens will be formed which can be easily visualised.
4. Read the band to observe against which of the viral proteins the antibody in the patient's serum has bound (Fig.18.1).

The Western Blot test is not a standardised test. Interpretation of bands depends on geographical locations. In Africa, for example, appearance of any two bands corresponding to any of the viral protein is regarded as positive.

Antibody against the Gag, P18, P24 and P55 appear first but decreases in titre with progression of HIV infection.

The ENV-specific antibodies – gp160, gp120 and gp41 persists in advanced stage of infection.

The capsid antigen p24 is usually detected before sero- conversion.

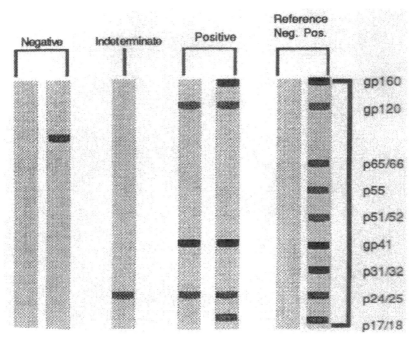

Fig 18.1 Western blot showing the presence of HIV-1 antibodies in bands corresponding to the HIV-1 antigens .

CD4 Count

The CD4 count helps predict the risk of progression of HIV infection and its complication. It is used in combination with the viral load test. The CD4+ count is used for determining the eligibility for antiretroviral drugs and assessment of response to the drug by the patient.

Procedure
Many companies now produce the needed reagents and protocols for CD4 count. Below is reproduced one of such protocols.

1. Add 20ul of whole blood from the patient to be tested to the test-tube.
2. Add 10ul of the CD45 monoclonal antibody which has been conjugated to human CD4. Again add 10 ul of CD4.
3. Mix gently and incubate at room temperature for 15 minutes.
Protect from light.
4. Add 400ul of no lyse buffer (Buffer A) and vortex gently.
5. Just before counting add another 400ul of buffer B. Perform a flow cytometry analysis to obtain the number of CD4 at an OD 488mm or 532.

A CD4$^+$ count of an HIV patient less than 200 is considered as having AIDS.

Viral Load

The viral load test is usually done alongside the CD4 count. It is used to:

1. Monitor response to ARV
2. Predict drug resistance
3. Predict disease progression
4. Decide whether to modify or change the ARV.

The viral load test measures the viral RNA copies per miltilitre of blood. There are three methods for measuring the viral load:-

(1) The polymerase chain reaction (PCR)
(2) The branched DNA method (bDNA) and
(3) The nucleic acid sequence based amplification (NASBA).

The PCR method will be briefly described here. Viral load determination of PCR takes the normal polymerase reverse transcription, amplification of target cDNA, hybridization of the PCR products to the probes and detection of probe bound amplified products.

Procedure

Specimen preparation

1. Collect blood in sterile tube with anticoagulant e.g. EDTA.
2. Centrifuge at 800 – 1600 x g for 20 minutes at room temperature to separate the plasma.
3. Store plasma in sterile tube at 2-8°C for 5 days.

It can be stored indefinitely at -70°C. Stored plasma should not be thawed more than three times.

A viral load test based on the principle of PCR is commercially available by the name AMPLICOR MONITOR. The procedure for specimen preparation, reverse transcription and amplification, detection and result are well described. The reader is advised to follow the manufacturer's instruction.

Further Reading

1. Cairns TM, Craven RC. "Viral DNA Synthesis Defects in Assembling Competent Rous Sarcoma Virus CA Mutants." *J. Virol 2001; 75: 242 – 250.*
2. Craven RC, Bennett RP, Wills JW. "Role of the avian retroviral protease in the activation of reverse transcriptase during virion assembly." *J. Virol 1991:65: 6205 – 6217.*
3. Fenyo EM., Monfeldt-Manson l., Chiodi F. et al. "Distinct Replicative and Cytopathic Characteristics of Human Immunodeficiency Isolates. *J. Virol 1988; 62: 4414-4419.*
4. Fitigerald ML, Vora AC, Zeh WA, et al. "Concerted Integration of Viral DNA Termini by Purified Avian Myeloblastosis Virus Integrase." *J. Virol 1992; 66: 6257-6263.*
5. Gibbs Jr CJ, Peters R., Graell M. et al. "Observation after human immunodefficient virus immunization and challenger of human immunodefficient seropositive and

seronegative chimpanzees." *Proc Natl Acad Sci, USA, 1991; 88:3348-3352.*

6. Hu WS, Temin HM. Genetic consequences of packaging two RNA genomes in one retroviral particle.: seudodiploidy and high rate of genetic recombination. *Proc Natl Acad Sci YSA 1990; 87; 1556-1560.*

7. Knipe. D.E. Lamb, R.A, Martin M.A., Roizman B. and Straus, S. *Fields Virology* 5th ed. Wolters Kluwer/Lippincott Williams and Wilkins. 2007 Philadelphia, PA

CHAPTER 19

Family CALICIVIRIDAE

To the family Caliciviridae belong two very important agents of acute gastroenteritis i.e. the Noroviruses and the Sapoviruses. The Norwalk virus is the prototype strain of these small round structured viruses known as Noroviruses.

They are small non-enveloped single stranded RNA viruses of positive sense genome with diameter ranging between 27-35nm. Noroviruses are the major cause of non-bacterial epidemic gastroenteritis in human, outbreaks usually occurring in families and communities. Both the noroviruses and sapoviruses have been incriminated in infant and young children diarrhea. Two other genera of the Caliciviridae are the Vesivirus of cat and the Lagovirus of rabbit.

Specimen Source and Sample Collection
Noroviruses can be detected in faecal sample and vomit us as well as contaminated water and food or fomites. Stool should be collected within the first 72 hours after onset of clinical signs.

Virus inoculation and isolation
None of the human caliciviruses has been adapted to cell culture. However the Vesivirus of feline can grow and form plaque in kidney fibroblasts. The Lagovirus will grow in primary rabbit hepatocytes.

A murine norovirus has been cultured in primary macrophage and dendric cells of murine origin.

Virus Identification

PCR

The PCR is the most widely used method for virus identification and diagnosis. This is because of the difficulty in growing the virus in culture. PCR will detect noroviruses in faeces and vomitus as well as contaminated food, water and fomites. The quantitative RT-PCR (q RT-PCR) also known as the real time PCR provides a rapid detection of the virus. For the PCR, the RNA must be highly purified and the primer must be specific for a particular strain. Sequencing can be used to determine geographical distribution and characterization of the various strains or genotypes during outbreaks.

Immunoassays

The discovery of the recombinant virus- like particles (r VLP) of the Noroviruses which are surrogates of the native virions in stool has led to the development of an antibody-based ELISA technique for the identification and diagnosis of noroviruses. Using norovirus specific and cross reactive monoclonal antibodies, the ELISA can detect viral antigens in clinical samples. The r- VLP antigen ELISA can also detect norovirus specific antibody. This can be used in large sero-epidemiological surveys.

Electron microscopy

EM will detect calicivirus directly from stools. The immune electron microscopy (IEM) is still more sensitive than the direct EM because very low quantity of the virus is usually found during the acute phase of the disease.

Further Reading

Atmar, R.L., Estes M.K. "Diagnosis of Noncultivatable Gastroenteritis Viruses, the Human Caliciviruses." Clin *Microbiol 2001:14 : 15-37.*

Cubbit WD. Jiang, XI, Wang J. et al. "Sequence Similarity in Human Caliciviruses and Small Round Structured Viruses." *Med Virol 1994; 43:252-256.*

Hale AD, TanakaT.N. Kitamoto N. et al. "Identification of an epitope common to genogroup 1 'Norwalk-like viruses' *Clin Microbiol 2000; 38: 1656-1660.*

Hang, X., Wilton M. Zhong W.M. et al. "Diagnosis of human caliciviruses by Use of Immunoassays." *J. Infect Dis 2000; 181: S349-359.*

Kageyama T., Kojima S., Shinohara M, et al. "Broadly reactive and highly sensitive assay for 'Norwalk-like viruses' based on real time quantitative reverse transcription –PCR." *Clin Microbiol 2003; 41: 1548-1557.*

Knipe. D.E. Lamb, R.A, Martin M.A., Roizman B. and Straus, S. *Fields Virology* 5th ed. Wolters Kluwer/Lippincott Williams and Wilkins.2007 Philadelphia, PA.

Madeley C.R. "Comparisons of the features of astroviruses and caliciviruses seen in samples of feces by electron microscopy." *Infect Dis 1979; 139: 519-523.*

CHAPTER 20

Family ARENAVIRIDAE

To the Family Arenaviridae belong those viruses that cause chronic infections in rodents. These rodents invade human habitats where, following virus shedding, the viruses infect humans and cause severe diseases.

All Arenaviruses are enveloped viruses with a bisegmented negative single stranded RNA genome. They are pleomorphic with size ranging from 40 to 200 nm in diameter. They cause some important human diseases, the severity of which may range from fatal haemorrhagic fever to neurologic aseptic meningitis. The most important of these diseases are the Lymphocytic choriomeningitis (LCM), the Lassa fever, Argentine haemorrhagic fever, Bolivian haemorrhagic fever, and the Venezuelan haemorrhagic fever etc. Only the Lassa fever virus will, however, be described in this book.

LASSA FEVER VIRUS

The story of Lassa fever cannot be complete without the mention of Laura Wine and Charlotte Shaws, the two American missionary nurses working in a remote hospital in Lassa village of the former Gongola State in the Northeastern part of Nigeria. These nurses were the first documented victims of this deadly virus that was first discovered in 1969. The virus is transmitted by the multimammate rodent, *Mastomys natalenses,(Fig.20.1)* found mostly in the savannas and forests of West, Central and East Africa. These rodents easily colonise homes where they set up the domiciliary circle of transmission. Lassa fever is characterised by fever, retrosternal pain, sore throat, cough, abdominal pain, vomiting, diarrhea, edema of the face, and mucosa bleeding. Deafness may result during the late stage of the disease.

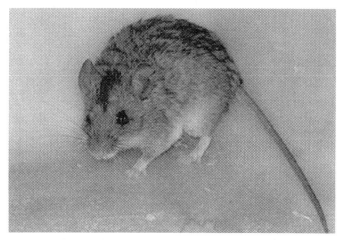

Fig. 20.1 The multimammate rodent *Mastomys natalenses*

Specimen source and sample collection

Blood or serum should be collected 14 days or more after onset of febrile phase. Necropsy tissues from post-mortem cases are also good source of specimens for virus investigation,

Extreme care should be taken while collecting samples. Personal protective equipments (PPE) must be used.

Virus inoculation and isolation

Lassa fever virus can be isolated from the blood, serum and post-mortem tissues in Vero cells. Virus inoculation should only be done in a BSC class 4.

Virus identification

Laboratory identification of Lassa fever virus can be done by the following laboratory methods.

IFA

Vero cell culture on immunohistochemical microscope slides can be stained by the direct method to detect and identify the virus. A known positive Lassa fever virus specific antibody must however be available. Lassa fever virus antibody can be detected by IFA using Lassa fever virus infected Vero cells as substrate.

ELISA

The virus antigen can be identified by capture ELISA in serum using known positive antibody conjugated to enzyme. This method is very reliable and simple to perform. Result can be obtained within 4 hours of testing. Lassa fever virus IgG and IgM can also be detected by ELISA in serum by the indirect ELISA technique.

CFT

The Complement Fixation Test can also be used to detect Lassa fever virus antibody is serum using Lassa fever virus –infected Vero cells as substrate.

PCR

The polymerase chain reaction is the most rapid diagnostic test for the identification of the virus. The test will detect viral RNA in the blood of patients.

Further Reading

1. Baush DA, Rollin PE, Demby AH, et al. "Diagnosis and clinical virology of lassa fever as evaluated by enzyme-linked imunosorbent assay, indirect fluorescent antibody test, and virus isolation." *J. Clin microbiol 2000; 38:2670 - 2677*

2. Demby AH, Chamberlain J, Brown DW, Clegg CS. "Early diagnosis of lassa fever by reverse transcription –PCR." *J. clin microbiol 1994, 32 (12) 2898 – 2903.*

3. Frame JD, Jahrling PB, Yalley – Ogunro JE, Monson MH "Endemic Lassa Fever in Liberia. II Serological and

virological findings in hospital patients." *Trans Roy Soc Trop Med 1984, 78 (5): 656 - 660.*

4. Johnson KM, Mccomick, JB, Webb PA, Smith ES, Elliott LH, King J. "Clinical virology of lassa fever in hospitalized patients J, *Infect Dis 1987, 155(3) :456 – 464.*

5. Trappier SG, Conaty AL, Farrar BB, AU, Perin D.D, McCormick JB, Fisher-Hock SP. "Evaluation of the polymerase chain reaction for diagnosis of lassa fever virus infection." *Am J Trop Med Hyg 1993;49 (2) 214-221.*

6. Wulff H, Lange JV "Indirect immunoflourescence for the diagnosis of lassa fever infection." *Bull World Health Organisation 1995:52(46):429-436.*

CHAPTER 21

HEPATITIS RNA VIRUSES

THE HEPATITIS VIRUSES

Viral hepatitis is a general term reserved for infections of the liver caused by one of at least six distinct hepatitis viruses. The viruses come from a wide range of virus families. Hepatitis A (HAV) is a picornavirus with positive single stranded RNA, hepatitis B (HBV) belongs to the Hepadnaviridae family, a double stranded DNA virus. HBV will be discussed under the DNA viruses. Hepatitis C (HCV) is a flavivirus, a positive single stranded RNA virus. Hepatitis E (HEV) is another single stranded RNA virus very close to the calicivirus. The fifth hepatitis virus is the Hepatitis D (HDV) which is often referred to as Delta agent. This is a circular RNA virus that is very much similar to a plant viriod. The sixth hepatitis virus is the recently discovered Hepatitis G virus (HGV).This virus is also referred to as GB virus- C (GBV-C).

HEPATITIS A (HAV) VIRUS

This virus is the cause of infectious hepatitis. The HAV has many similarities with the other picoraviruses in terms of morphology and structure but differs significantly from these viruses in its nucleotide and amino acid sequences, absence of CPE in cell culture and resistance to temperatures that will normally inactivate other picornaviruses.

There is only one serotype of HAV. The incubation period is about 15-40 days and the onset is sudden. Appearance of anti-HAV IgM coincides with appearance of clinical symptoms. Presence of only anti-HAV 1gG is an evidence of past exposure and immunity.

HEPATITIS C VIRUS (HCV)

HCV is the first Non A Non B (NANB) hepatitis agent discovered after the HAV and HBV and this was made possible as a result of the refinement of powerful and sensitive molecular biological techniques of the 1980s. HCV is a flavivirus, an enveloped icosahedral positive strand RNA virus.

The HCV RNA contains two major capsid proteins, the E1 and E2 and a central region protein, the P7 and NS2. The remaining part of the polyprotein contains the non-structural proteins, NS3, NS4 and NS5.

HEPATITIS D VIRUS (HDV)

The HDV is highly defective virus. It cannot produce infective virions without the help of a co-infecting helper virus. The Hepatitis B virus supplies the HBsAg protein which the HDV requires for reinfection and which it acquires during budding. The RNA encodes only one single protein, the Delta antigen which complexes with the RNA. The RNA is single stranded negative sense.

HEPATITIS E VIRUS (HEV)

Hepatitis E virus is a non-enveloped positive stranded RNA virus very close to the calicivirus. Like the HAV, it is enteric by transmission, hence it is often referred to as enteric Non A Non B (ENANB) hepatitis. HEV is characterised by an indefinite surface structure that is slightly different from the calicivirus. It is easily distinguishable from the smooth featureless surface of HAV.

HEPATITIS G VIRUS (HGV)

Hepatitis G virus, also known as GB virus – C (GBV-C) was discovered in 1995. It is a single stranded RNA virus belonging to the Flaviviridae family as HCV with which it is genetically similar. It causes mild disease in human and is not known to cause serious liver damage like other hepatitis viruses. Hepatitis G virus is commonly found in association with HIV. About one third of people infected with HIV are likely to be co-infected with HGV.

Sources of specimens and collection

Stool and serum are the preferred specimens for virus identification and diagnosis. Liver biopsy specimens can also be used.

Virus Inoculation and Isolation

HAV

HAV will grow in some primary or continuous cell lines of primate origin. Primary African Green Monkey Kidney (AGMK), primary human fibroblast and continuous human diploid lung cell (MRC5), Vero, BS-C1, fetal rhesus monkey kidney FRhK4, FRhK6, human hepatoma cell, PLC/PRF/5 have all been used for propagating HAV. However, there is usually no viable cytopathic effect. Viral multiplication can only be detected indirectly using other immunological assays like IF, IEM, or molecular techniques such as RT-PCR or Hybridisation test for direct HAV RNA detection

Virus Identification

Serological test provides the best means of HAV identification.

Immunflourescnce test
The immunofluorescent technique can be used to identify HAV in liver biopsy.

ELISA

The ELISA technique will detect anti-HAV IgM in serum of patient with recent acute infection. ELISA will also detect the total anti-HAV antibodies which measure both the IgM and IgG antibodies. The total anti HAV test determines the immune status of an individual following immunisation.

Hepatitis C Virus (HCV)

Virus isolation and identification.

HCV can be isolated in cultured mammalian cells such as peripheral blood mononuclear cells and primary hepatocytes from human and chimpanzees. Because there is no visible CPE, RT-PCR can be used to detect virus replication. Identification is by serology and direct detection of viral RNA.

Enzyme Immunoassay

Anti HCV IgM in serum or plasma can be detected by ELISA to establish initial infection.

Nucleic Acid Testing(NAT).

This test is used to confirm the serological test and also to determine the genotype. The HCV –RNA test is a direct indication for on-going HCV replication.

Hepatitis D Virus (HDV)

Virus Isolation and Identification

No cell lines, including those derived from human liver, are susceptible to HDV infection. HDV is always associated with HBV. HBsAg, HBeAg and HBV DNA will always be found in the serum of HDV infected patients. The HDV is identified by both serological and molecular test.

ELISA.

An ELISA technique can detect anti HDV in serum. Presence of IgM anti-HDV confirms recent infection. Hepatitis D virus antigen will appear in the serum which is followed by the appearance of IgM anti HDV and IgG anti HD.

PCR
Early identification of HDV infection is detected by RT-PCR. This method has overcome the limitation of serological detection of HDVAg.

Hepatitis E Virus (HEV)

Virus Isolation and Identification

There is no efficient cell culture system for the isolation of HEV. Because of this reason, serological test plays an important role in the identification and diagnosis of HEV. Test for anti HEV-IgM and IgG are available commercially. A rising titre of 1gG anti HEV identifies the virus.

RT-PCR detects HEV nucleic acid in the blood and feaces in the acute phase.

HGV

Virus isolation and identification
The virus, like the HCV, has been shown to replicate in human peripheral-blood mononuclear cells. Blood and serum are the best sources of specimen. The virus does not produce any visible CPE and therefore identification can only be confirmed by serology or RT-PCR or direct RNA detection. It must however be differentiated from HCV

Further Reading

1. Bradley D.W., Maynard J.E., Hindman S.H. "Serodiagnosis of viral hepatitis A: detection of acute-phase immunoglobulin M anti hepatitis A virus by radioimmunoassay."*Jour Clin Microbiol 1977; 5:521-531.*

2. Costa –Matiolli M, Di Napoli A. Ferre V. et al. "Genetic variability of hepatitis A virus." *J Gen Virol 2004; 84:3191-3201*

3. Knipe. D.E. Lamb, R.A, Martin M.A., Roizman B. and Straus, S. *Fields Virology* 5th ed. Wolters Kluwer/ Lippincott Williams and Wilkins.2007 Philadelphia, PA

4. Koziel MJ, Peters MG. "Viral hepatitis in HIV infection." *N Engl J Med 2007; 356: 1445-54.*

5. Locanini S.A. Ferris A.A. Lehmann N.L. "The antibody response following hepatitis A infection." *Intervirology 1977; 8 309-318*

6. Yotsunayagi H. Iino S.Koike K. et al. "Duration of vireamia in human hepatitis A viral infection as determined by polymerase chain reaction." *J Med Virol 35-40.*

DNA VIRUSES

CHAPTER 22

Family ADENOVIRIDAE

The adenovirus was first isolated from the adenoid tissue from where the virus derived its name. Since that first isolation, adenoviruses have been isolated from various organs of patients where they cause a variety of clinical syndromes like pharygoconjunctivitis, acute febrile pharyngitis and keratoconjunctivitis and infantile gastroenteritis in humans. However, more adenoviruses have been isolated in chimpanzees, monkeys, reptiles, dogs, and chickens. At present there are about 51 human serotypes which are distinguished by neutralisation test. Each adenovirus replicates better on the tissue of their natural host. The 51 serotypes are grouped into six subgroups on the basis of their ability to haemagglutinate red blood cells. Type 3, 7, 11, 14 and 16, 21, 34, 35 and 50 will haemagglutinate monkey erythrocytes while Types 1, 2, 5 and 6 will haemaggltinate rat erythrocytes completely. Types 8, 9, 10, and 26 will haemagglutinate human type O-erythrocytes.

Structurally, the adenoviruses are about 70-100nm in diameter with each virus particle consisting of 252 capsomeres. They are icosahedral in symmetry. On the surface are 240 hexons and 12 pentons. The pentons are attached to fibers.

All adenoviruses, except those of avian, produce a group specific antigen which can be detected in a complement fixation test.

Specimen source and collection

Specimen collection will depend on the clinical manifestation of adenoviral infection. For respiratory symptom, throat swabs, nasal swabs should be collected. For keratoconjunctivitis and other ocular infection, eye swabs or eye wash are the best to collect. Rectal swabs and stools should be collected in suspected adenoviral enteric infections.

Specimen should be collected from affected site at such a time as to optimise viral isolation and to detect antigens and NA directly. These periods are usually between 1-3 days at the time of acute respiratory infection, 3-5 days from nose, throat, stool, eye and as long as 2-12 months or even longer in urine, stool, throat of immunocompromised patients.

Virus inoculation and isolation

Adenovirus are best isolated in cells of human origin. Human embryo kidney (HEK) cells are the best for all groups of adenoviruses, although established cell lines like HEp-2, HeLa, KB and A549 cell lines are very sensitive and will easily support the growth of adenovirus. The A549 is derived from lung adenocarcinoma while the KB is of nasopharyngeal carcinoma origin. Clinical specimens obtained from throat swabs, nasal washes, conjunctival swabs can be kept frozen at -70°C before inoculation.

Adenovirus CPE is characterised by rounding and swelling which aggregate into grapelike clusters. Some adenoviruses can grow in the polio specific cell line, L20B, where the CPE can be easily differentiated from the usual rounding type of CPE observed with enteroviruses.

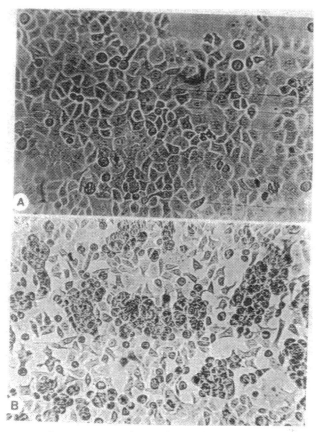

Fig.22.1 Adenovirus cythopathic effect in HEp-2 cell line
A. Uninfected HEp-2 B. HEp-2 infected with adenovirus type 3
Reproduced by permission from G. D. Hsiung Diagnostic Virology,
Yale University Press,1982.

Virus identification

Adenovirus from infected cell can be harvested by 2-3 cycles of vigorous freeze-thawing. Both infected cultured cells and fluid should be harvested because of the cell-associated nature of the virus.

Cytopathology of infected cells
Adenoviruses produce adenovirus-specific intra nuclear basophilic Feulgen-positive inclusion bodies when stained in heamotoxylin-eosin or feulgen reaction.

Complement Fixation Test

All the human adenoviruses possess a group specific antigen which is the product of the viral hexon. Preliminary identification can be made using the CFT. A known reference serum must however be available for the definitive identification.

Immunofluorescence Technique

The ability of adenovirus infected cell antigen to cross react with adenovirus reference antiserum makes the immunofluorescent technique a useful and simple technique for preliminary identification.

The IF and the CFT cannot be used to identify serotypes. However a type-specific monoclonal antibody used to differentiate serotype 40 and 41 have been developed and can be used in IF and ELISA.

Haemagglutination Inhibition Test

Specific adenovirus serotyping can be done using the haemagglutination inhibition test. Viruses initially identified in CFT or IF can be tested for haemagglutinating property using different types of erythrocytes. Serotype can be confirmed by using specific monoclonal antibodies to inhibit the HA.

ELISA

The ELISA technique can be used to directly detect adenovirus antigen from respiratory, ocular or stool samples.

The Meridian Biosciences Inc. has developed a kit Adenoclone which can detect mostly all human serotypes. Because this method is less sensitive, a negative result must be confirmed by cell culture.

Molecular Technique

The polymerase chain reaction (PCR), quantitative real time PCR and restriction enzyme digestion of the viral DNA are also used for virus identification. These methods are however not used routinely for diagnostic purposes.

Neutralization Test

For those serotypes like type 18 and 31 that will not haemagglutinate any type of RBC, neutralisation test in tissue culture must be done using type-specific antiserum.

Serodiagnosis.

The CF, HA, HI, serum neutralisation and ELISA can be used to detect antibody response to adenoviruses. The CFT recognises the group hexon antigen. A single CF antigen detects responses to many adenoviruses serotypes. A four-fold rise in CF antibody signifies current infection.

Further Reading

1. Herrman JF, Peron-Henry D.M. Blacklow N.R. "Antigen detection with monoclonal antibodies for the diagnosis of adenovirus gastroenteritis Infect."*Dis 1987;155:1167-1171.*

2. Hierholzier JC, Halonen P.E. Dahlen P.O. et al. "Detection of adenovirus in clinical specimens by polymerase chain reaction and liquid-phage hybridisation quantitated by time resolved fluorometry." *Clin Microbiol 1993; 31: 1886-1891.*

3. Hitt, M, Bett A, Prevec L et al. Construction and propagation of human adenovirus vectors In: Celis J.E eds. Cell Biology: A Laboratory Handbook vol. 1, San Diego Acad Press 1998

4. Hsiung GD, Caroline KY, Fong and Marie L. Landry. *Hsiung's Diagnostic Virology* 4th ed. Yale University Press 1994.

5. Kassel J.A. Adenoviruses In: Lenette EH, Schmidt NJ. eds. Diagnostic procedures for viral, Rickettsial and chlamydial Infections. Washington DC American Public health Association. 1979: 229-256.

6. Knipe. D.E. Lamb, R.A, martin M.A., Roizman B. and Straus, S. *Fields Virology* 5th ed. Wolters Kluwer/Lippincott Williams and Wilkins.2007 Philadelphia, PA

CHAPTER 23

Family HERPESVIRIDAE

The viruses belonging to the herpesviridae family are all morphologically similar sharing the same architecture. But serologically and biologically they are distinguished into eight herpesvirus groups infecting humans. These are Herpes simplex 1,Herpes simplex 2, Varicella-Zoster (V-Z), Epsein Barr virus, Cytomegalovirus (CMV), Human Herpes virus – 6, Human Herpes virus – 7 and Karposi Sarcoma-associated Herpesvirus. Recent classification of the family have further divided the family into three subfamilies -

Alphaherpesvirinae (Simplexvirus, varicella zoster virus)
Betaherpesvirinae (Cytomegalovirus, Roseolovirus HHV- 6) and
Gammaherpesvirinae(EBV and HHV-8)

Herpesvirus has been isolated from other lower animal species like non-human primates, horses, dogs, pigs, cats etc and birds as well as from fishes.

The herpesviruses are linear double stranded enveloped DNA viruses with an icosahedral capsid of about 125nm in diameter with 162 capsomeres. They share one significant biological property among themselves, which is latency in their natural hosts which often manifests in form of recurrent disease when equilibrium between the host and the virus is lost. This may be brought about by adverse environmental conditions like cold and stress. The herpesvirus infections present in a variety of clinical manifestations ranging from simple fever blisters or cold sores to a generalized infection of children as seen in chicken pox or cytomegaly. Virus multiplication occurs in the nucleus of infected cells forming intranuclear inclusion Cowdry type A inclusion bodies.

THE ALPHA HERPESVIRUSES

HERPES SIMPLEX VIRUS

Sources of specimens and collection

Specimen for laboratory diagnosis depends on clinical manifestation of the infection. Skin scrapes, cerebrospinal fluids, stool, urine and throat swabs, nasopharyngeal swabs and conjuctival fluids can be collected depending on the clinical manifestation. Specimens should be collected and inoculated immediately. In infants with hepatitis or other gastrointestinal complication, duodenal aspirates can be collected. Clinical specimens should be transported on ice.

Virus inoculation and isolation
Virus Isolation remains the most important test for confirmation of Herpes simplex virus infection.
The virus will grow in a variety of tissue culture cells including both primary and established cell lines from human and non-human origin such as Vero, HEp-2, RK, HEK, HEF and HeLa. A 0.2ml of viral suspension inoculated into any of these cell lines will show CPE within 3-5 days. However CPE appears more rapidly in RK and therefore tend to be the cell of choice for the isolation of the virus. The growth of the virus in RK can be used to differentiate between the human herpes from other HSV viruses because the human viruses seldom grow in non-primate cell lines. CPE is characterised by rapid cellular degeneration where they may form clusters. HSV will form good plaques in cell culture.

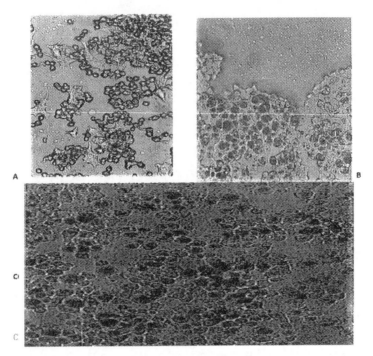

Fig 23.1 Herpes simplex virus cytopathic effect in Hep-2 cell line (A) Diffused . (B) Focal.*(C)* **Uninfected.** *Anthony A. Oni et al. Isolation of Herpes Simplex virus from Sexually Transmitted Disease patients in Ibadan, Nigeria. Dept of Virology, College of Medicine, University of Ibadan, Nigeria*

Virus Identification

1.   Immunofluorescent staining

HSV 1 and 2 can be rapidly identified both in lesions and in infected tissue culture by the indirect IF staining using specific HSV monoclonal antibody. This technique can be used to differentiate HSV from Varicella-Zoster and cytomegalovirus.

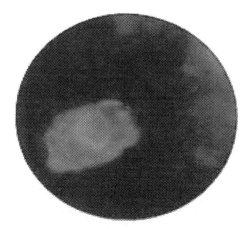

Fig 23.2 HSV-infected epithelia cell from skin lesion

2.   Neutralisation or plague reduction neutralisation test (PRNT)
HSV-1 and HSV-2 can be identified and typed by using neutralisation
test or plaque reduction neutralisation test. Type specific antiserum to
each of the virus must be used. The antiserum that inhibits or causes
about 80% or more plaque reduction is indicative of the HSV isolate.
Because of antigenic cross reactivity, neutralisation test may not
correctly differentiate between HSV- 1 and HSV-2.
HSV-1 can be differentiated from HSV-2 by plaque selectivity in
Guinea pig embryo cell (GPE) and chicken embryo fibroblast (CEF).
HSV-1 will form plaque in GPE but not in CEF, while HSV-2 will
form plaque on both GPE and CEF.

3.   Cytologic examination of cells
Cytologic examination of cells from the cervix, mouth, skin,
conjunctival or corneal lesions is often useful in the identification of
HSV infection. Cellular scrapings of the lesions should be smeared
on a slide and fixed in cold ethanol and stained according to the
method of Papanicolaou or Giemsa. The presence of intranuclear
inclusion bodies and multinucleated giant cells are suggestive of HSV
infections.

Serological identification

The most commonly used serological test for HSV diagnosis and identification is the complement fixation test (CFT), passive haemagglutination test, neutralisation test, immunoflorescent and ELISA.

Molecular Method

The PCR method has been very useful for the diagnosis of HSV encephatitis and skin lesions. Primers from the DNA sequence common to both HSV-1 and HSV-2 are used in PCR to detect HSV DNA in CSF of patients suspected of having HSV encephalitis.

VARICELLA-ZOSTER VIRUS

Varicella-Zoster virus (VZV) is the cause of chicken pox in children during primary infections. The diseases is characterized by fever and a generalised, pruritic vesicular rash. VZV exhibits latency after primary infection, the reactivation of which gives rise to herpes zoster called shingles in adulthood.

Sources of Specimens and Collection

The most reliable source of specimen for VZV isolation are fluids from the vesicle and swabs obtained from the lesions. VZV is heat labile and specimen should be inoculated fresh and immediately.

Virus inoculation and isolation

Varicella-zoster virus can be isolated in cells of human fibroblast origin like WI-38 and human fetal diploid cells. VZV does not cause CPE in cells other than those originating from humans.

Inoculated cell culture may show CPE between 5-7 days, much slower than what is observed in HSV. VZV will not show CPE in RK as compared to the rapid CPE caused by HSV in this same cell line.

Virus Identification

Immunoflorescence Assay

Immunofluorescent staining can be used to identify varicella-zoster virus in infected cells or lesions. A type-specific antiserum conjugated to the fluorescein must however be available. The method provides a rapid diagnosis.

Molecular technique
Varicella-zoster RNA can be detected directly from tissues or infected cells by PCR.

Serology
Assays for detection of antibodies to varicella zoster virus are very useful for the determination of immune status of subjects either after vaccination or following exposure.
A number of sensitive tests are available. The most sensitive test is the fluorescent antibody membrane antigen assay (FAMA).
The indirect FA and the dot-ELISA (d-ELISA) and the membrane – ELISA (M-ELISA) have been found to be equally sensitive for the measurement of varicella zoster virus IgG.

BETAHERPESVIRUSES

Betaherpesviruses comprise cytomegalovirus(CMV) and the Human herpesvirus virus HHV-6A and HHV-6B variants. The (CMV) is associated with opportunistic disease. CMV is readily isolated from variety of mammals. Tissue distribution of the virus in diseased host follows a definitive pattern. They exhibit species specificity and only particular type of cells is susceptible within a species. The CMV is characterised by enlargement of the infected cell (cytomegalia). CMV infection is of particular interest in pregnant women and women of child bearing age. The virus has been associated with mononucleosis where it can cause severe organ damage. The virus will also cause congenital abnormalities in newborns.

Specimen source and sample collection

Urine, saliva and genital secretions are the specimens of choice for CMV isolation and identification. Serum can also be collected for serology and viral DNA detection by Real-Time PCR.

Virus Inoculation and Isolation

Human CMV can be isolated only on cell lines of human origin such as W1-38, human diploid fibroblast (HDF), human embryonic lung, or foreskin fibroblast monolayers. CMV is characterised by slow growing focal CPE which may take between 2-3 weeks to appear. Rapid isolation and recognition of the virus in tissue culture can be achieved by the enhancement of infection method.

This is done as follows:

Procedure
1. Infect monolayer with the prepared clinical sample.
2. Allow virus to absorb for 3-4 hours at 37°C.
3. Incubate further for 12-24 hours at 37°C in maintenance medium.
4. Freeze-thaw the monolayer at two cycles.
5. Perform a low speed centrifugation to pellet the cells.
6. Using CMV-specific monoclonal antibody, detect the immediate early antigens in the cells.

This enhancement method allow for rapid isolation of CMV in tissue culture.

Virus Identification

CMV is easily identified in stained urine sedimentation by the appearance of cytomegalovirus particles. CMV identification is often based on the slow growth in tissue culture, specific organ cytopathology and limited susceptibility to cell culture. CMV pp 65 antigen can be easily detected in the nuclei of peripheral blood neutrophils (Fig.23.3).

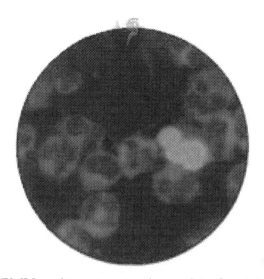

Fig. 23.3 CMV pp65 antigen in the nuclei of peripheral blood neutrophils

Serology
Neutralisation test, complement fixation test (CFT) and Immunohistochemical method (IFA) are used to detect antibody rise in serum. The CFT is the most common and more convenient. An ELISA technique for the detection of antibody and CMV antigen is available. This is more sensitive and will detect antibody to most of the viral proteins earlier than the other serological tests.

pp65 Antigenemia Assay
This assay is used for detection and quantitation of CMV in the blood of immunocompromised patients using a non-culture method. It uses monoclonal antibody to detect the tegument protein pp65 in the peripheral blood leucocytes by the immunostaining of cytocentrifuge preparation of blood cells.

Result is expressed as pp65 positive white blood cells (WBC) per 200,000 counted. The number of pp65 +ve WBC correlates with the risk of the disease. The antigenemia assay is simple to perform with commercial kits now available.

HUMAN HERPES VIRUS 6 AND 7

Human herpesvirus 6 and 7 (HHV-6, HHV-7) share some common properties with the CMV virus. They grow mainly in T-lymphocytes, although they can also infect other cell lines. There are two variants of HHV-6 – A and B. HHV-6B is the cause of exanthema subitum (ES) in infants and is characterised by rash, diarrhea, cough, enlargement of the lymph node, bulging of the frontales, fever and neurological symptoms and mononucleosis-like infection in adult. Primary infection with HHV-7 is similar to that of HHV-6, but the frequency is, however, lower.

Source of specimen and collection

Peripheral blood mononuclear cells (PBMC) are the specimen of choice for HHV-6, but saliva can also be collected for HHV-7. Blood must be collected within the first 7 days for the virus to be detected in blood.

Virus inoculation and isolation

HHV-6 will grow in a variety of human cells such as matured CD4$^+$, natural killer cells (NK), primary fetal astrocytes, dendritic cells and PBMC. HHV-6A grows better in cultured cells of neuronal origin than HHV-6B. HHV-6B produces little CPE while HHV-6A produces productive lytic infections.

For successful isolation of the virus in these cell lines the PBMC must be activated by PHA and maintained in medium containing IL-2. CPE characterised by refratile giant cells will appear within 7-10 days after co-culture with lytic degeneration of the cells.

Virus Identification

Serology

IFA: This is the most commonly used serological method for the identification of the virus. Infected cells can be used as the source of the antigen, while a known positive reference antiserum must be available to confirm identification.

ELISA
Direct and indirect ELISA techniques are available and they are more sensitive than the IFA and immunoblot. The immunoblot is however more specific.

Other serological methods such as neutralisation and radioimmunoprecipitation are also used for virus identification. Antibody avidity test can be used to identify most recent infection.

Molecular Method
The PCR is used to detect HHV-6 and HHV-7. DNA multiplex primers and other primers for the rapid identification of HHV-6 variants and simultaneous detection of HHV-6 and HHV-7 and for all the HHV are all available. The DNA can be detected in the blood of exanthema subitum (ES) patients during the acute phase.

Detection of HHV-6 in serum by PCR is significantly important for diagnosing active infection.

EPSTEIN BAR VIRUS (EBV)

This is the causative agent of infectious mononucleosis characterised by mild transient fever, pharyngitis, lymphadenopathy and general malaise. It has been associated with Burkit and Hodgkins lymphomas.

The presence of the virus can be demonstrated by cultivation of lymphocytes from infectious mononucleosis patients.

Serological tests are the best method for identification of the infection in the laboratory.

Serological diagnosis
The Immunofluorescent staining techniques will detect the various EBV antigens in cells. The marmoset cells line B95-8, B95a is easily transformed by the virus, and demonstration of the virus by immunostaining in these cells is an indication of EBV infection. The differentiation of virus-specific antigens and the development of corresponding antibodies are indicative of the status of EBV infection.

Further Reading

1. Anderson NE, Powell KF Croxson MC. "A Polymerase chain reaction assay of cerebrospinal fluid in patient with suspected herpes simplex encephalitis." *J. Neurol. Neurosurgery Psychiatry 1993; 56:520-525.*

2. Boeckh M, Bowden RA, Goodrich JM, et al. "Cytomegalovirus antigen detection in peripheral blood leukocytes after allergenic marrow transplantation." *Blood 1992; 80: 1358-1364.*

3. Braun DK, Dominguez G, Pellett PE. "Human herpesvirus 6." *Clin Microbiol Rev 1997; 10: 521-567.*

4. Cardinali G, Gentile M, Cirone Metal. "Viral glycoproteins accumulate in newly formed annulate lamellae following infection of lymphoid cells by human herpes virus 6." *J virol 1998; 72:9738-9746.*

5. Caserta MT, Hall CB, Schnabel K et al. "Primary human herpes virus infection: A comparison of human herpes virus 7 and human herpes virus 6 infections in children." *J Pediatr 1998; 386-389.*

6. Chou J, Roizman B. "The terminal sequence of the herpes simplex genome contains the promoter of a gene located in the repeat sequences of the L component." *J virol 1986; 7:629- 637.*

7. Dobson AT, Sederati F, Devi - Rao G, et al. "Identification of the latency - associated promoter by expression of rabbit beta- globin mRNA in mouse sensory nerve ganglia recombination herpes cimplex virus." *J virol 1989; 65 :3844 – 3851.*

8. Kemp W, Adams V, Mirandola P, et al. "Persistence of human herpesvirus 7 in normal tissues detected by expression of a structural antigen": *J Infect Dis. 1998; 178: 841-845.*

9. Pereira L, Maidji E, McDonagh S, etal. "Insight into viral tramsmission at the inter-placental interface." *Trends Microbiol 2005; 13(4): 164-174.*

10. Rowley A, Lakeman F, Whithey R, et al. "Rapid detection of herpes simplex virus DNA in cerebrospinal fluid of patients with herpes simplex encephalitis." *Lancet 1990; 335:440 - 441.*

11. Tanaka K, Kondo T, Tongoe S, et al. "Human herpes virus 7: another causal agent for roseola (exanthema subitum)." *J. Pediat 1994; 125: 1-5.*

12. Troedle - Atkains. J, Demmler GJ, Buffone GJ. "Rapid diagnosis of herpes simplex virus encephalitis by using the polymerase chain reaction." *J. Pediatr 1993;123:376-380.*

CHAPTER 24

Family HEPADNAVIRIDAE

HEPTATITIS B VIRUS (HBV)

The hepatitis B virus (HBV) belongs to the Hepadnaviridae family, a double stranded DNA virus consisting of an outer lipid envelop and an icosahedral nucleocapsid core enclosing the viral DNA. HBV is the agent of serum hepatitis. The virus in its chronic infection form has also been found to cause liver cirrhosis and hepatocelluar carcinoma in some infected hosts. This virus was discovered by Blumberg et al. from an Australian aborigine when it was initially referred to as the Australian antigen but now named hepatitis B surface antigen (HBsAg). The virus exists in three forms, the Dane particles which are actually the virion particle, the surface antigen, HBsAg and the filamentous form of about 22 nm in diameter.

The HBV is a DNA virus with an envelope. Unlike all other enveloped viruses, the HBV is relatively stable to organic solvents. It is also heat and pH-resistant. The genome is surrounded by the core antigens (HBcAg and HBeAg). On the surface lipid bilayer is the surface antigen (HBsAg) i.e. the Australian antigen. The presence of these antigens plays important diagnostic roles in the determination of the status of the disease.

Persistent presence of HBsAg in the blood after acute infection is a sign of transition from acute to the chronic form of the disease.

Loss of HBsAg is an indication of complete elimination of the virus. Presence of anti-HBsAg antibodies is a mark of protection. HBeAg is a serological marker of active viral replication while loss of circulating HBeAg and appearance of anti-HBe antibodies often indicate the end of active viral replication, but the beginning of clinical recovery from infection.

The HBcAg is the major nucleocapsid protein. Appearance of anti HBc IgM is an indication of current acute infection. This is replaced by anti-HBc IgG which persists for a very long time.

Sources of specimens and collection

The HBV can be detected in serum semen and virginal fluids. However serum is the preferred specimen of choice for virus identification and diagnosis if the patient is alive. Liver biopsy specimens can also be used, especially after death.

Virus inoculation and isolation

Hepatitis B virus is not easily grown in tissue culture. However the virus can be successfully grown in human peritoneal macrophages after about 14-21 serial blind passages. The virus will not show any visible CPE but isolation can be detected by positive HBc, HBe, and HBs antigens using either ELISA, CFT or IFT tests. The virus has also been successfully isolated in human adult hepatocytes after about 10 weeks of serial passages. Like in the human macrophages, the virus will not show any characteristic CPE but can be detected by a positive HBcAg.

Virus Identification

The various antigens and antibodies produced during HBV infection provide good blood markers for the easy identification of the virus in clinical specimens.

Like HAV, serological test is the best for virus identification and diagnosis. A very efficient ELISA technique for the identification of the various markers is readily available in most laboratories.

HBsAg
Persistence of the surface antigen indicates chronicity while loss is an indication of elimination of the virus.

Anti-HBsAg
This is a marker of protection. The appearance of anti HBs antibody is either a sign of past infection or immunisation.

HBeAg
Presence of HBeAg in the serum is a sign of active viral replication. Loss of this antigen and appearance of anti-HBeAg signify end of viral replication and beginning of clinical resolution.

HBcAg
Appearance of anti HBc IgM is the first sign of acute infection, especially if found in combination with HBsAg. Evidence of coexistence with HDV is done by checking for HDVAg and anti-HDV 1gM.

Assay for viral load
This is the best method for determining the presence of circulating virus.

Viral DNA can be detected by RT-PCR and the number of virions per ml of serum can be calculated. The viral load PCR assay is also used to assess infection status and also monitor response to treatment.

The algorithm for the diagnosis of Hepatitis A, B,C, and D is shown in Fig.24.1

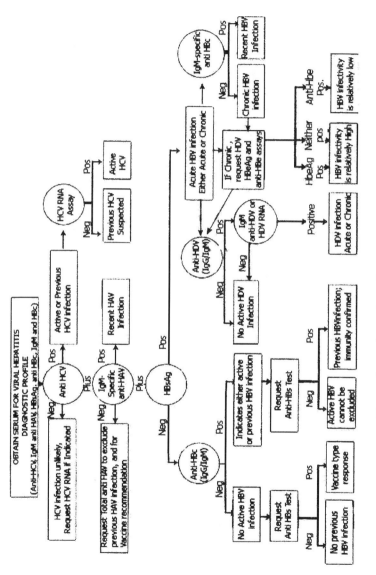

Fig. 24.1. Algorithm for the diagnosis of Hepatitis A, B, C and D viruses.

Further Reading
1. Blumberg BS, Alter HJ, Visnich S. "A "new" antigen in leukemia." *JAMA 1965; 191: 541-546.*
2. Chu C.J., Hussain M, Lok A.S. "Quantitative serum HBV DNA levels at different stages of chronic hepatitis B infection." *Hepatology 2002; 36:1408-1415.*
3. Hsiung GD, Caroline KY, Fong and Marie L. Landry. *Hsiung's Diagnostic Virology* 4th ed. Yale University Press 1994.
4. Knipe. D.E. Lamb, R.A, Martin M.A., Roizman B. and Straus, S. *Fields Virology* 5th ed. Wolters Kluwer/Lippincott Williams and Wilkins.2007 Philadelphia, PA
5. Lok A.S. McMahon B.J. "Chronic hepatitis B." *Hepatology 2001; 34: 1225-1241.*
6. Milan N. Milovanovic, Zera Vivanovic-Marinkovic et al. "Hepatitis B virus in tissue culture system." *Intervirology, Vol 27,No1. 1987; 1-8.*

CHAPTER 25

Family POXVIRIDAE

The Family Poxviridae comprises the variola virus, the agent of small pox – a once dreaded human virus that always leaves its mark in every population where it strikes. Small pox had been eradicated globally since 1977. The Poxviruses are divided into two sub families-Chordopoxvirinae and Entomopoxvirinae. The Chordopoxvirinae comprises such viruses like Cowpox virus, Ectromelia, Vaccinia, monkeypox and Variola viruses. Poxviruses infect a variety of hosts like birds, pigs, sheep and goats. However, the human poxviruses are found in these genera- Orthopoxvirus, Parapoxvirus, Yatapoxvirus and Molluscipoxvirus. Majority of the human poxviruses are zoonoses except variola and molluscum contagiosum that are solely human. Only Vacccinia and Cowpox viruses will be described in detail here.

VACCINIA AND COWPOX VIRUSES

There is no natural host for vaccinia virus and the origin of the virus is unknown. However variants of the virus are known to infect other animal species apart from humans.

Cowpox virus has a wide range of hosts with cattle as the predominant host. Infections in cattle are sometimes limited to the teats and the udder. The virus causes localised lesions in humans.

Source of specimen and sample collection

Skin scrapings, fluids from the vesicles as well as the skin crusts are the best sources for virus isolation.

Virus Inoculation and Isolation

Vaccinia and cowpox viruses can be readily isolated in a variety of primary and established cell lines. Cell lines such as Vero, HEp-2C and Monkey kidney are susceptible to the virus. Virus suspension should be inoculated directly into monolayer cells The pox viruses are relatively stable at room temperature, and therefore virus may be kept for a time before inoculation.

The embryonated egg is the most reliable and sensitive system for virus inoculation and isolation. Virus suspension should be inoculated into the chorioallantoic membrane of 12-14 day old embronated egg and incubated at 36-38°C. Laboratory animals such as rabbit and baby mice can also be inoculated with viral suspension. The virus suspension should be inoculated into the rabbit intradermally while the mouse is inoculated intracerebrally.

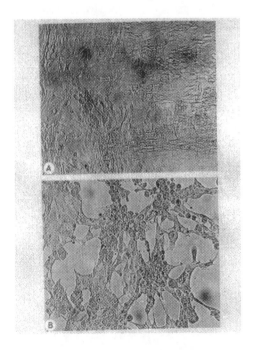

Fig.25.1 Vaccinia virus cytopathic effect in RhMK cell culture (100X). (A) Uninfected cell. (B) Cell infected with vaccinia virus *(Adapted by permission from G.D.Hsiung Diagnostic Virology, third edition, Yale University Press 1982).*

Virus Identification

Direct staining

Because of the specific morphology and the unique size of the poxviruses, presumptive identification can be made by direct negative staining of the vesicular fluid by electrom microscopy (EM).

Smears of scraping can also be stained by Giemsa. Virus infected tissue culture cell can also be stained by the immunofluorescent technique provided there is a known positive immune serum.

Stains of the infected cell will show eosinophylic intracytoplamic inclusion bodies (Downie Bodies in Cowpox and Guarneri Body in Vaccinia).

Morphological observation of virus pock growth on CAM can be used to identify the viruses. The CAM will show large diffused haemorrhagic necrotic spots or lesions.

PCR

A good polymerase chain reaction system has been developed for the direct detection of the viral genomes in skin lesions, scrapings and tissue culture infected cells.

Further Reading

1. Damon I. Esposito J.I. Poxviruses that infect humans. In: Manual of clinical microbial 8th ed. Murray PJ Baron EJ eds Washington DC ASM Press 2003;1583-1597.

2. Hammanlund E. Lewis M.W. Carter S.V. et al. "Multiple diagnostic technique identifies previously vaccinated individuals with protective immunity against monkeypox." *Nat Med 2005;11(9):1005-1011*

3. Hsiung GD, Caroline KY, Fong and Marie L. Landry. *Hsiung's Diagnostic Virology* 4th ed. Yale University Press 1994.

4. Karem K.I. Reynolds M. Braden Z. et al. "Characterization of acute phase humoral immunity to monkeypox: use of immunoglobulin M enzyme-linked immunosorbent assay for detection of monkeypox infection during the 2003 north American outbreak." *Clin Diagn Lab Immunolog 2005; 12(7): 867-872.*

5. Knipe. D.E. Lamb, R.A, Martin M.A., Roizman B. and Straus, S. *Fields Virology* 5th ed. Wolters Kluwer/Lippincott Williams and Wilkins.2007 Philadelphia, PA

6. Meyer H.Damon I.K. Esposito J.J. "Orthopoxviruses diagnostics." *Method Mol Biol 2004; 269:119-134.*

7. Olson V.A. Laue T. Laker M.T. et al. "Real- time PCR system for detection of orthopoxviruses and simultaneous identification of smallpox virus." *Jour Clin Microbiol 2004;42(5);1940-1946*

CHAPTER 26

Family PARVOVIRIDAE

The Parvoviridae are small non-enveloped viruses with single stranded DNA genome, icosahedral in symmetry with a diameter of between 20-25 nm. They are the smallest of the DNA viruses. The family is divided into two subfamilies-the Parvovirinae and the Densovirinae. The Parvovirinae infects mostly vertebrates and are found in five different genera i.e. the Parvoviruses, Erythroviruses, Dependoviruses, Amdoviruses and the Betaparvoviruses. All the viruses except the Dependoviruses are autonomous. They do not require co-infection with a helper virus to produce infection.

The Parvoviruses infect a variety of animals such as mice, rat, canine, chickens, rabbit, bovine and equine. In those cases where the virus is not autonomous, they are often associated with a helper virus, mostly adenovirus and are called Adeno-Associated virus (AAV). They can also be associated with the herpesvirus.

Canine parvovirus is a virus of veterinary importance causing disease in young puppies with high mortality especially in unvaccinated dogs. The disease is characterised by enteritis.

HUMAN PARVOVIRUSES

The most significant human Parvoviruses are the B19 virus and the associated erythroviruses. The B19 parvovirus is the cause of erythema infectiosum, an acute biphasic illness in children characterized by transient aplastic crisis especially in patients with hemolymphadenopathy. In adults, the disease is associated with flulike symptoms, fever, malaise, myalagia, polyathritis and artthralgia. However the most obvious sign is skin rash.

B19 is transmitted by respiratory secretions but infection can also be through contaminated blood products.

Source of specimen and sample collection

Serum, bone marrow, cord blood, amniotic fluid, fetal ascites, urine, and throat swabs are the best sources of specimens for virus isolation and identification. Serum should be collected during viremia and aplastic crisis in patients with haemoglobinopathy.

Virus isolation

B19 Parvovirus can be isolated in some special cell lines such as suspension culture of erythropoetin stimulated human erythroid bone marrow cells, haemopoetic cells from human fetal cells and cells from human cord blood. Virus isolation is, however, not a routine clinical practice for identification of the virus.

Virus identification

Antigen/antibody detection

Parvovirus specific antigen can be detected in clinical samples by the method of counterimmunoelectrophoresis (CIEOP) and antigen capture ELISA.

The appearance of rash coincides with the appearance of Parvovirus specific IgM in serum, followed a few days later by appearance of IgG. Therefore both IgM and IgG can be detected by antibody capture ELISA. This method is sensitive and specific. However, for both the CIEOP and ELISA tests, Parvovirus monoclonal B19 specific monoclonal antibody must be used in order to confirm the tests.

Electron Microscopy

Electron microscopy (EM) and immuno-electron electron microscopy (IEM) can be used to visualise and identify the virus. For the IEM, specific antibody or monoclonal antibody must be used to facilitate detection.

Molecular Method

Both the probe hybridisation technique and the polymerase chain reaction (PCR) have been used to identify the B19 virus. These methods are particularly useful when serum antibody is not available in an immunodefficient patient or when the virus can not be isolated in any of the cell cultures.

Further Reading

Knipe. D.E. Lamb, R.A, Martin M.A., Roizman B. and Straus, S. *Fields Virology* 5th ed. Wolters Kluwer/Lippincott Williams and Wilkins.2007 Philadelphia, PA.

CHAPTER 27

Family POLYOMAVIRIDAE

The Polyomaviruses are small DNA viruses which multiply efficiently in cells of their host origin to produce cell death but produce a transforming or oncogenic infection in other species. They are non-enveloped, double stranded circular DNA viruses of 40-45 nm in diameter. The polyomaviruses are resistant to heat and formalin. They replicate in the nucleus of host cells. They infect a variety of mammalian and avian species. Polyomaviruses are the causes of two important human diseases – the JC and BK, named after the initials of first patients from whom the viruses were first isolated. JCV was isolated from the brain of a Hodgskin's lymphoma patient with progressive multifocal leucoencephalopathy (PML) while BK was isolated from the urine of a renal transplant recipient. Both viruses cause human disease by active infection of their target cells which is the brain for JCV and the kidney and bladder for BKV. JCV is characterised by neurological sypmtoms which may include muscle weakness, gait disturbance, hemiparesis subcortical dementia, sensory and visual deficits. BKV is associated with kidney disease and cystitis, and in some cases, pneumonia and encephalitis.

Sources of specimen and sample collection

Brain and CSF are the best sources of sample for JCV while urine is the best for BKV. Two or more CSF samples should be collected within a period of 2 weeks.

Virus Inoculation and Isolation

Although JCV can be grown in cell culture, it takes about 6-31 days with several blind passages for any visible effect to develop.Virus isolation is not routinely practised for identification. Both viruses can be grown in primary fetal glial cells (PHFG), but BKV is much easier to grow. It can be easily grown in other cell lines such as human primary epithelial cells, primary human embryonic kidney and lung cells, human foreskin fibroblast, Vero and CV-1

Virus identification

The advancement in molecular diagnostic techniques has made the identification of the polyomaviruses much easier. Virus isolation is difficult and may not be too helpful.

Antigen and genome detection
JCV DNA and antigen detection will give a definitive identification and diagnosis of the virus. Specific monoclonal antibodies are available for both JCV and BK polyomaviruses.
PCR can be used to detect viral genome in the brain tissue and CSF. This method has proved very sensitive and specific. PCR will detect BKV in urine. The presence of decoy cells (renal epithelial cells) in urine is an indication of active BKV infection.
BKV can be identified by the immunohistochemical method using immunoflourescent or immunoperoxidase staining of tissue for T-antigen. Specific monoclonal antibody to the virus must however be available. The viral DNA can also be detected by the nucleic acid hybridisation.

Electron microscopy
The polyomaviruses can be easily identified under the electron microscope. The viruses are scattered in the nuclei of the infected

cells. The EM is an important tool for the final identification of the polyomaviruses.

Serology
Antibody to polyomaviruses is wide spread. Serology may not be very useful in assessing infections. However, antibody to polyomaviruses can be measured by the haemagglutination inhibition test or the ELISA.

The Simian vacuolating virus (SV40)
The Simian vacuolating virus, SV40, is the polyoma virus of primate, primarily monkey. The virus was first isolated from cell culture of African green monkey kidney that had been used for the production of poliovirus vaccine. The virus produces no cytopathic effect in rhesus monkey cells. The SV40 is one of the most studied viruses as model system for understanding transcription, DNA replication, RNA processing, and oncogenic transformation. The cloning of SV40 genome ushered in the era of recombinant DNA research. SV40 is used as vector for vaccine and gene delivery vehicles.

Further Reading
1. Carter JJ, Koutsky LA, ltughes JP, et al. "Comparison of human papillomavirus types 16, 18 and 6 capsid antibody responses following incident infection." *J infect Dis 2000; 181;1911-1919.*
2. Dillner L. "The serological response to papillomaviruses. Semin. Cancer." *Biol 1999;9;423-430.*
3. Doorbar, J, "The papillomavirus life cycle." *J Clin Virus 2005; 32(suppl f); 57-515.*
4. Hedquist BC Bratta I, Hammarin AL, et al. "Identification of BK virus in a patient with acquired immune deficiency syndrome and bilateral atypical retinitis." *Ophthalmology1999; 106:124-132.*
5. Major EO, Amemiyak, Tornattore CS et al. "Pathogenesis and molecular biology of progressive multifocal leukoencephalopthy; the virus-induced denyelinating

disease of the human brain." *Clin Microbial Rev. 1992; 5;49-73.*

6. Voltz R, Jagir G, Seelosk, et al. "BK virus encephalitis in an Immunocompetent patient." *Arch Neurol 1996;53; 101-103.*

7. Sweet, BH, Hilleman MR. "The vacuolating virus, SV40." *Proceedings of the Society for Experimental Biology and Medicine. 1960; 105:420-427.*

CHAPTER 28

Family PAPILLOMAVIRIDAE.

The Family Papillomaviridae comprises a group of non-enveloped epitheliotropic DNA viruses that induce benign lesions of the skin (warts) and the mucous membrane (condylomas). They have also been implicated in epithelial malignancies such as cancer of the cervix and other tumors of the urogenital tracts. The papillomaviruses are small viruses with diameter between 50-55 nm. They possess an icosahedral shape and they replicate in the nucleus of the epithelia cells. The virion particle is a double-stranded circular DNA surrounded by a capsid of 72 capsomeres.

There are about 60 types of human papillomaviruses based on epidemiological classification. The study of papillomaviruses became prominent after their link with cervical and other anogenital cancers.

The papillomaviruses are difficult to grow in tissue culture because they replicate only on stratified squamous epithelia which is very difficult to reproduce in culture. Clinical identification of the virus has been made possible by techniques such as PCR and molecular hybridisation that are able to identify the viral DNA. The distribution of the various papillomavirus types and their clinical features is shown in Table 28.1.

Genital warts caused by the human papillomaviruses are the most common form of sexually transmitted disease while cervical cancer is the most important cancer attributable to human papillomaviruses. Depending on their risk of progression to malignancies, the various types of papillomaviruses can be categorised into high, intermediate and low.

High   -   HPV Types 16, 18, 45 and 56
Intermediate -   HPV Types 31, 33, 35, 51, 52, 58,
Low   -   HPV Types 6, 11, 42, 43, 44.

Sources of specimen and collection

Cervical swabs, biopsy samples from cancer cells, cell scrapings from the female genital tracts are the best sources of clinical samples for viral detection. Samples should be collected in 1 ml volumes of Pap transport medium. These are available commercially.

Virus isolation

Isolation of papillomaviruses in tissue or laboratory animal is difficult. They have not been successfully adapted to any cell line since they only replicate in squamous epithelial cells which are difficult to mimic *in vitro*.

Virus identification

Identification of human papillomaviruses has been done by those techniques which detect viral DNA or RNA in samples.

Viral Antigen Detection

Because human papillomaviruses have not been grown successfully in tissue cultures, very few reagents are available for antigen/antibody detection of the viruses. A broad spectrum cross reactive immune serum specific for the genus and prepared by inoculating bovine papillomavirus into rabbit has been used to detect from tissue sections capsid antigen using the immunoperoxidase staining technique. The limitation of this technique is that it can only detect the antigen in productive lesions and not in high grade dysplasia and cancers.

Molecular method

A PCR technique utilising consensus primers in conjunction with reverse line blot assay for specific hybridisation has been developed. A synthetic RNA probe that is capable of capturing the viral DNA is also in use. Real time PCR is also a very useful molecular technique for the identification of the virus genomes.

The hybrid capture II test which is capable of detecting the high risk types is the only test currently licensed.

The development of HPV –based assays for screening in clinical practice has substantially reduced incidences of cervical cancers. These HPV –based assays may, in no distant future, replace the Pap smear screening.

DNA/RNA detection

Sensitive and reproducible molecular assays have been developed to detect human papillomavirus DNA and RNA in cervical swabs and biopsy samples.

Electron microscopy

The papillomaviruses can be directly visualised in clinical specimens by the negative staining or thin section technique.

Serology

A few serological assays based on ELISA format and neutralisation that monitors antibody response has been developed. However, these tests lack the sensitivity and specificity to make them useful as routine clinical diagnostic tests.

Skin	Cutaneous warts	1,2,3,4,7,10,26,27,28,29,37,38,41,46,48,49.
	In association with epidermodysplasia verruciformis	5,8,9,12,14,15,17,19,20,21,23,233,24,25,36,47,50.
Genital tract mucosa	Condylomaacuminatum, cervical carcinoma,etc	6,11,16,18,31,33,34,35,39,,40,42,43,44,45,51,53,54,55,56,58
Oral cavity mucosa	Focal epithelia hyperplasia	13,32
Other sites		30,57.

Table 28.1 Clinical manifestation of the
various human papillomavirus types.

Further Reading

1. Carter J.J. Koutsky L.A. Hughes J.P. et al. "Comparison of human papillomavirus type 18, 16 and 6 capsid antibody responses following incident infection." *Infect Dis 2000; 181: 1911-1919.*

2. Denny L.A. Wright Jr T.C. "Human papillomavirus testing and screening." *Best Pract Res Clin Obstet Gynaecol 2005; 19: 501-515.*

3. Dillner J. "The serological response to papillomaviruses." *Semin. Cancer Biol 1999;9;423-430.*

4. Doorbar J. "The papillomavirus life cycle." *Jour Clin Microbiol 2005;32 [Suppl 1]: S7-S15.*

5. Knipe. D.E. Lamb, R.A, Martin M.A., Roizman B. and Straus, S. *Fields Virology* 5th ed. Wolters Kluwer/Lippincott Williams and Wilkins.2007 Philadelphia, PA .

6. Richart R.M. Barron B.A. "A follow-up study of patients with cervical dysplasia." *Am. Obstet Gynaecol 1969:105: 386-393.*

INDEX

of reovirus in nonprimate kidney, 183

of rubella in rabbit kidney cell, 192

of vaccinia in RhMK cell, xiii

D

Dane particles, 252
delta antigen, 229
dengue haemorrhagic fever (DHF), 208
dengue shock syndrome (DSS), 202, 208
deoxynucleotides (dNTPs), 113-14
deoxyribonucleic acid (DNA), 6, 9
dextran separation method, 28
diethanolamine buffer, 89
double immunodiffusion, 55

E

Earle's Balanced Salt Solution, 44
Ebola haemorrhagic fever, 199
Ebola virus, 199
echoviruses, 136, 156
electroimmunodiffusion, 63
electron microscopy (EM), 222, 262, 265
end point, determination of, 101-2

enteric non-A non-B (ENANB) hepatitis, 229
enteroviruses, 136-37, 140-41, 158
enzyme linked immunosorbent assay (ELISA), 87-88, 92, 141, 147, 151
ephemerovirus, 196
epitopes, 57-58, 62, 158, 188
Epstein-Barr virus, 249
erythema infectiosum, 261
ethidium bromide, 120, 148
exanthema subitum (ES), 248-49

F

feline immunodeficiency virus (FIV), 213
fetal calf serum (FCS), 21, 34, 44
Ficoll-Hypaque, 27
filoviruses, 199-201
flaviviruses, 202, 205
fluorescein isothiocyanete (FITC), 80
Fungizone, 29

G

Gag precursor, 214
GB virus-C (GBV-C). See hepatitis viruses: hepatitis G
gelatin, 21, 29
gel comb, 120

intraperitoneal inoculation, 37-38

intratypic differentiation, 141, 147-49

J

Japanese encephalitis, 202

jaundice, 203

JC, 264

K

kaolin treatment, 72

Kaposi's sarcoma-associated herpesvirus, 240

Karber formula, 104

keratoconjunctivitis, 235-36

kidney cell culture, preparation of, 47

L

laboratory
  accreditation, 16
  manual, 15
  safety, 16
  staff, 15

Laemmli loading dye, 98

lagovirus, 221

Lassa virus, 224-26

lentivirus, 213

leucocytes, 28, 165, 247

lymphocytes, 27-28, 126-27, 165, 249

lymphocytic choriomeningitis (LCM), 224

M

macrophages, 127, 176, 215, 253

male sterility, 172

Marburg haemorrhagic fever, 199

Marburg virus, 199

Mastomys natalensis, 224

measles virus, 64, 164-68

  RBC preparation for, 66

methyl cellulose overlay, 107

molecular serotyping, 140, 158

monoclonal antibodies, 83, 88, 97, 126, 127-30

morphological subunit, 9

multinucleated giant cells, 166, 243

mumps virus, 172-73

Murray Valley encephalitis, 202

myeloma cells, 126-27

  fusion of lymphocytes and, 130

N

National Institute of Public Health and Environment (RIVM), 146, 155

natural killer cells (NK), 248

Negri bodies, 197

neuraminidase, 164, 169, 178

red blood cell (RBC)
 day-old chick, 194
 guinea pig, 170-71, 179-80
 human group O, 65, 184-85
 monkey, 65, 68
red blood cells (RBC), 235
Reed and Muench, method of, 105
regulatory bodies, 13-14, 16
reoviruses, 185
respiratory syncytia virus, 173-74
retrovirus, 213
reverse transcriptase (RT), 147, 213
rhinoviruses, 136, 160-62
ribonucleic acid (RNA), 6, 9
rinderpest virus, 176
RNA extraction, 116
RNAse free water, 117
RNase inhibitor, 124
rotaviruses, 186-89
rubella virus, 190-95

S

sera treatment, 71
serological assay, 53-54, 270
serum, 44-45
Shaws, Charlotte, 224
signaling lymphocytic activation molecules (SLAM), 165
simian immunodeficiency virus (SIV), 213
specimen processing, 26-27
sputum, 27

stains
 Coomassie brilliant blue, 99
 crystal violet, 107
 Giemsa, 243, 259
 methyl blue, 107
 neutral red, 107
 Papanicolaou. See Pap smear screening
 phosphotungstate acid (PTA), 187
 silver, 99
standard operating procedure (SOP), 14
St. Louis encephalitis, 202
stool, 21, 26, 138, 184, 187-88, 230, 236
stool treatment, 26
substrate buffer, 89
suckling mice, 139, 209
supraoptimal temperature, 150
swabs
 nasopharyngeal, 179, 241
 rectal, 21, 138, 236
  throat, 138, 172, 179, 184, 191, 236, 241, 262
SYBR Green, 122
syncytia, 36, 215

T

Taq DNA polymerase, 115, 124
TEMED, 99
tissue culture infective dose (TCID), 102
tissues